From State Hospital
to Psychiatric
Center

From State Hospital to Psychiatric Center

The Implementation of Planned Organizational Change

Murray Levine
State University of
New York at Buffalo

Foreword by
Yoosuf A. Haveliwala, M.D.
Creedmoor Psychiatric Center

LexingtonBooks
D.C. Heath and Company
Lexington, Massachusetts
Toronto

RC
445
.N68
L48

Library of Congress Cataloging in Publication Data

Levine, Murray, 1928-
From state hospital to psychiatric center.

Bibliography: p.
1. Psychiatric hospital care—New York (State) 2. Community mental
health services—New York (State). 3. Organizational change. 4. Harlem
Valley Psychiatric Center (N.Y.) I. Title.
[DNLM: 1. Hospitals, Public—Organ—New York. 2. Community mental
health centers—Organ—New York. WM28 AN6 H2L6f]
RC445.N68L48   362.2'2'0684   80-779
ISBN 0-669-03810-5

Copyright © 1980 by D.C. Heath and Company

Published simultaneously in Canada

Printed in the United States of America

International Standard Book Number: 0-669-03810-5

Library of Congress Catalog Card Number: 80-779

To my wife, Adeline,
whom I first met in a mental hospital,
and who has been
my personal community support system for
lo these many years.

Contents

Foreword

Americans are fascinated with change. Technological change, self-improvement, national growth, and personal growth represent strong values within American national character. Yet despite the strong ideology in favor of change, many of America's large organizations and institutions are marked less by their evolving character than by stasis.

For all practical purposes, prior to July of 1974, Harlem Valley Psychiatric Center was a custodial state mental hospital, an example of an institution in stasis. A rural, residential mental hospital, it provided good, clean housing and three square meals a day, while protecting its patients from harm. The hospital grew as more and more patients from metropolitan New York were sent far from the city into more serene rural counties, in keeping with the practices of the early part of this century. Harlem Valley was an asylum in the country. Its structure, its goals, and many of its personnel fitted the static character of a traditional custodial organization.

Harlem Valley changed significantly after July of 1974. The changes illustrate how a mental-health institution can alter its organization, its goals, and its treatment modalities, how it can change from a custodial hospital to a modern, comprehensive mental-health center. This book describes how the changes were accomplished.

The Harlem Valley Psychiatric Center operated within the constraints normal to service institutions embedded within a state-government bureau. Although its problems may seem to differ on the surface from those of other types of organizations, I believe the institutional issues and the problems I faced are common to all organizations. Consequently, the work accomplished at Harlem Valley provides data meaningful for the comparative study of organizations. By looking past the mental-health context, one can discern the deep structure of change.

Change in a governmental system is extremely difficult. Bureaucratic systems are structured to maintain stability. Statutes and regulations control the system, while the state's budgetary practices and procedures set parameters for change. The civil-service system regulates but also limits personnel changes. I had a good grasp of these issues because of my experience within the state system. I believe changes were accomplished successfully because I learned to take advantage of the rules and regulations or bend them when necessary to effect the changes I had in mind. It was not necessary to break any law or to violate any regulation. It takes a certain skill to understand and to use the rules to bring about change in what appears to be a rigid bureaucracy. In fact, this skill may be the critical factor in successful leadership in such settings, the skill and the willingness to accept calculated risks.

Prior to becoming director of the Harlem Valley Psychiatric Center, I worked in one of the newly founded community-mental-health centers. I was impressed by the philosophy and the organizational structure of the new center. I quickly developed the desire to try to change an older custodial institution into a newer and what I believe to be superior practice. I sensed the challenge, but I believed it could be done, for it was clear that changes would have to be accomplished by reallocating the same resources. Existing dollars would have to be pushed in new directions since new dollars were simply not available. But the goal was worthwhile. I thought then, and still think, that the changes improved the quality of mental-health care by bringing into being a more comprehensive network of services. Although the challenge was to my administrative and leadership abilities, the desire to produce change was deeply rooted in my firm belief that patients and their families would benefit.

While there is an accumulated body of knowledge that strongly suggests that proper care for the mentally ill should be provided in the communities in which patients live, organizations do not alter their philosophies of care and their styles of operation simply because of new knowledge. People do not appreciate change and especially not rapid change. Preparation for change is a necessary part of any plan for change. But it is also true that professionals trained in new knowledge acquire a zeal to implement their service ideas. Thus, even within a traditional, custodial hospital, the seeds of change lay dormant, waiting for leadership to provide the organizational climate for the seeds to grow and develop.

When I was appointed director of the Harlem Valley Psychiatric Center in July of 1974, the effective statewide institutional grapevine resulted in my reputation preceding my physical presence. My philosophy of mental-health care, my views of state-hospital organizations, and my youth were major elements creating an air of expectancy in which the changes I had in mind could be initiated. As chief executive officer, I knew I had to be the primary driving force behind the reorganization process. I knew the process would be facilitated by developing a "Zeitgeist" or a spirit of change, and by bringing in personnel who wholeheartedly supported the new directions. These were critical steps, for I was working in a government bureaucracy, an agency long characterized by stasis.

In assuming the role of director, I knew that all my actions had to fall within the raison d'etre of the institution: Harlem Valley Psychiatric Center existed to serve the mentally ill. I wanted to change a custodial hospital, but all the organizational changes could be justified only within an explicit philosophy, firmly held, of providing better care. In this case, to change the system meant to develop a network of community services first so that patients released from the hospital would continue to be served and not thereby become the victims of change.

In contrast to some proponents of community-based services who feel that funds will somehow magically follow patients into communities, I firmly believe that the dollars and the resources associated with these dollars (namely, necessary manpower and a network of community services) must precede the patients into the community. If funds follow patients, then for all practical purposes a budgetary cycle of one or more years would have to run before services could evolve for patients already released into the community. Patients cannot wait for such budgetary considerations. The most critical period for any patient newly released from a mental hospital is the first three to six months. Patients must receive services immediately upon their return to the community.

As chief executive officer, I faced the dilemma of how to provide services in the community without new funds and while maintaining in-hospital services. I accomplished the task, aided by my executive group, by using the flexibility inherent in the budgetary and bureaucratic state-hospital system. For example, during the annual budgetary cycle, when we had staff openings, we hired people to work in the communities rather than placing them on the inpatient services. Of course, to do this we had to find some initial "fat" in the system. But there was not much fat, and we had to reach some compromises. Inpatient services were already thinly staffed, and funds were limited. The compromise consisted of reducing the budget for institutional care and hiring staff to work in the new community-based services.

I reduced the budget for inpatient services by closing two wards within the hospital and transferring those patients to other wards. There was some overcrowding in a few wards, but the move provided flexibility to transfer existing staff from the closed wards as well as to hire new staff to work in the network of community services that we could then develop rapidly. Overcrowding the wards slightly, and temporarily, was not hazardous from the point of view of safety or proper care. An increased workload of one or two patients in each of the 60 wards of a hospital did not affect programming significantly, since the custodial wards provided little beyond routine care. An overload of one or two patients could not have had a deleterious impact. But whatever inconvenience resulted, the slight overcrowding lasted only a few months. Once community-based services were in place, patients were released from the hospital into the care of our own community-based staff. Ward censuses dropped drastically, in turn increasing the opportunities to redeploy staff and to develop additional services.

Some patients resisted the change process. They had learned to live in a familiar environment and did not want to be released into a community from which they had been isolated for years. They considered such changes threatening. The unfamiliarity of the new situation made some anxious. Staff members were critical in providing support and in helping patients overcome their fears. But many staff members were also anxious about their job situations and their job security, which made our task even more difficult. Moreover, while patients and staff resisted change, we also had to face resistance to change from the community. People were concerned about the release of mental patients. There were charges that the hospital just wanted to reduce its census and save money and was thus "dumping" its patients.

One of the earliest organizational problems, then, was dealing with the various forms of resistance. Patients were my first concern. We concentrated our efforts on winning over even the most recalcitrant of patients. We encouraged those who saw value in community living to talk with fellow patients and explain the advantages from their point of view. We took patients to various community facilities to show them the positive side of community living—the flexibility of the programs, the convenience, and especially the increased freedom. We assured them that ward staff with whom they had developed close relationships would visit and help them adapt to living within a community setting.

One of the most effective elements of change was the new group of community-oriented professionals who gradually filled the ranks of our staff. This group of people, both in the inpatient services and in the outpatient community settings, believed in community-based mental-health care. Their dedication and enthusiasm built a rapport with the patients and helped convince most that it was to their advantage to live outside the hospital.

We dealt with staff resistance by outlining how the hospital's move toward community-based mental-health care would provide even greater job security. Over the decade prior to 1974, the institution had been continuously threatened by budgetary-minded people in state government as well as by key legislators who had often spoken of closing Harlem Valley because it had no function in the new scheme of care. I presented the staff with the concept that making Harlem Valley into a model institution, in fulfillment of the Department of Mental Hygiene's long-standing policy of moving to community-based care, would demonstrate the hospital's relevance. Some of the staff understood what I was saying.

We provided the staff with opportunities for training in community mental health. Early on, we started a community-mental-health nursing-training program. Many paraprofessionals enrolled as students. The administration provided release time for their training at no financial cost to the staff member. We developed relationships with community colleges and other academic institutions so that we could offer relevant courses on the hospital grounds. We offered higher civil-service grades and higher salaries as incentives for those who participated in college programs and who worked toward attaining higher academic qualifications.

To deal with actual and potential staff resistance, we brought workers from the community services back to the hospital to talk with inpatient ward staff about the services offered in the outpatient settings. Similarly, we took ward staff to the community clinics and day hospitals to talk with their outpatient colleagues and to witness for themselves their former patients' progress. This aspect of our program was a major factor in reducing staff resistance. Staff were reassured that their former patients were receiving good care in the community.

Community resistance had to be met in other ways. We embarked on a public-education campaign in order to demonstrate that Harlem Valley Psychiatric Center was not engaging in the practice of "dumping" patients. We went public. We participated in various community board meetings and local mental-health councils. We publicly stated that our outpatient services were not restricted to the hospital's ex-patients but would be available to the community at large. Patients who were still functional and productive in a psychiatric sense, and their families, were brought into the hospital's service network and helped to continue to live in the community. Through their participation, we developed an advocacy group for each of our community-based programs. Such efforts contributed to the softening of community resistance.

It is important to discuss how I was able to accomplish these changes within the constraints of a relatively large bureaucratic organization. I believed that I could not accomplish the task by acting unilaterally as an authoritarian chief executive. An executive committee, composed of professional mental-health personnel and administrators, had to develop into a decision-making body. It became regular practice for all decisions to be made by this executive body acting as a group, with open discussion among its members and the chief executive officer. I resisted making decisions based on private conversations between myself and a staff member. I insisted that the decision-making process go on in the executive committee in an open and public manner. Consequently, suspicion, rumors, and discontent were kept to a minimum. On occasion, I would disagree with the executive committee's recommendations. I was responsible for the hospital's management, and therefore I chose to act as a chief executive officer in the final sense of that term. However, I followed a personal rule of always discussing the basis for my decision and opening the issue (and myself) to feedback and criticism before a decision was made final.

The executive committee's minutes were distributed widely. Members of the executive committee sought feedback from their staffs. We instituted a system of monitoring in order to check the effects of our decisions. If any errors were uncovered, we had a direct communication link by which we could assess the need for correction and make it quickly. The involvement of staff helped to broaden the director's constituency, for the executive committee identified itself with the changes and the decisions. The director was not a lone actor, but rather he became the senior member of an executive team.

Finally, I wish to draw the reader's attention to the fiscal impact of the changes. No extra funds were provided to help Harlem Valley Psychiatric Center accomplish the tasks of deinstitutionalizing and developing a network of community-based services. Harlem Valley Psychiatric Center was not chosen by higher authorities in New York State to become a demonstration project or to exemplify fulfillment of the state's policy goals. However, the results described in this book did serve as examples, both in leadership and in mental-health services, of what could be accomplished through local initiative.

Despite a 25-percent inflation rate in the five years from 1974 to 1979, the institution's budget decreased by 25 percent. At the same time the number of patients served by the institution more than doubled, increasing staff productivity considerably. The doubling occurred as a result of three factors: First, all patients who continued with the hospital inpatient programs remained under the care of the institution; second, all patients who left the inpatient hospital system were transferred into the outpatient system; and third, new patients were enrolled from the community.

The total number of patients served increased. There were 1,800 inpatients in 1974, but in 1979 there were only 500 inpatients and 3,500 outpatients. More patients were provided more services with a smaller and tighter budget. Yet— and this is an accomplishment of which I am most proud—the quality of care in the hospital as a whole improved tremendously. In 1974, for example, the hospital's inpatient staff-to-patient ratio was one staff member for every two patients. In 1979, we brought that ratio up to one staff member for every one patient, thereby doubling the amount of professional and paraprofessional manpower available for patient care.

Quality of care improved in other ways as well. Our staff frequently saw patients who were discharged, in our community clinics, in our day programs, and in our sheltered workshops, making for a continuity of care difficult to achieve otherwise. Using the same financial resources, we broadened our community-support system from practically zero in 1974 to the point where our comprehensive-care program was designated in 1978 as a site for a federal demonstration program. We extended services to all members of the community and made available, 24 hours a day, seven days a week, mobile crisis-intervention teams staffed with professionals, including psychiatrists.

In short, our efforts resulted in regaining and maintaining full accreditation from the Joint Commission on Accreditation for Hospitals, even though standards for that accrediting body became higher and higher during that five-year period.

What has happened to my beliefs since the changes were accomplished? I am even more convinced now that it is possible to improve the quality of mental-health care and to make large bureaucratic organizations such as state hospitals more responsive to the demands of changing mental-health needs and knowledge. I believe that in the short term as well as the long, the changes at Harlem Valley Psychiatric Center were beneficial to patients and were cost-effective. Programs that work for the benefit of patients and yet remain within the constraints of reasonable budgets can be developed, monitored, and modified as necessary. It was that philosophy and approach that enabled us to provide a modern system of comprehensive mental-health care under the aegis of a state hospital.

Our goal is the best quality of care. The Harlem Valley experience proves convincingly that organizational change leading to an improved quality of care can be accomplished within the constraints of present budgets (assuming, of course, that present budgets are not hopelessly inadequate, as they are in some places). It takes no special outlay of additional funds to accomplish the task. I believe that maximum changes are possible even within rigid bureaucracies and that constructive changes can be made by using funds that are presently being spent less productively.

Yoosuf A. Haveliwala, M.D.
Creedmoor Psychiatric
Center

Acknowledgments

This study was completed under contract between the New York School of Psychiatry, which was assisting the New York State Office of Mental Health in implementing a demonstration grant under the National Institute of Mental Health-sponsored State/Local Community Support System Demonstration and Replication Project, and Human Services Research and Planning, Inc., Buffalo, New York. The author is indebted to Dr. Yoosuf A. Haveliwala, his executives and staff at Harlem Valley, and the many individuals who participated in interviews or provided documentary materials for their cooperation. Ms. Louise Hubbard, then of the Harlem Valley staff, was most helpful in arranging for visits, in suggesting people to interview, in making documents available, and, in general, in facilitating the study in every way. I am particularly appreciative of the help provided by Mike Ross, now with the New York State Office of Mental Health, who was then project officer for the New York School of Psychiatry. The comprehensiveness of this report owes much to Mike's insistence that all bases be touched. It also owes much to his astute criticism of an earlier draft. Don Lund, of the Office of Mental Health, provided significant assistance to the project. My colleagues at the State University of New York at Buffalo and at Human Services Research and Planning, Frank Baker, Doug Bunker, Ray Hunt, and Drew Hageman, John Northman, and Mark Ramsdell, read and criticized portions of the manuscript and contributed valuable ideas and observations. Finally, I want to thank Lee Ann Pawlick and Erma Rawlings, who effectively and efficiently translated scribbled-over first drafts into clean error-free copy.

1 Introduction

The Harlem Valley Psychiatric Center, a New York State institution, located in Wingdale, a rural community, changed within a period of four years from an old-line, predominantly custodial institution to a modern psychiatric center. The events to be described in this case study of organizational change began in 1974 and continue at this writing, although the case study itself covers the period from 1974 to 1978. The psychiatric center, under the leadership of its director, Dr. Yoosuf A. Haveliwala, reduced its inpatient census rapidly, developed an elaborate network of outpatient and after-care services, and reduced its admission rate as well. All this was accomplished with a declining budget, and by means of reallocating resources rather than by adding new ones to its budget. This case study describes how the change was accomplished.

Harlem Valley's program and its agenda were very much in keeping with the dominant thrust of national mental-health policy as reflected in the report of the congressionally appointed Joint Commission on Mental Health and Illness (1961), President John F. Kennedy's Message to the Congress on Mental Illness and Mental Retardation (5 February 1963), and the Community Mental Health Centers Acts of 1963 (PL 88-164), 1965 (PL 89-105), and subsequent amendments through 1975. Bloom (1977) and Foley (1975) provide descriptions and summaries of the legislation and the politics of passing the bills. As Levine and collaborators (Levine et al. 1981) point out, federal mental-health policy has had a rather consistent direction since the end of World War II.

President Kennedy's 1963 Message to Congress, the first presidential message devoted exclusively to the problem of mental-health services, called for a halving of the state-hospital population within a decade. It also called for the development of an elaborate network of community-based services to prevent hospitalization and to provide continuity of care for those who were discharged from hospitals.

The federal thrust reflected long-standing problems with the state-hospital system. When the first state hospital opened in Worcester, Massachusetts, in 1830, there was great optimism about what the new moral therapy, developed in Europe by Pinel and Tukes, could accomplish. Indeed, in their first few years, excellent results were reported (Bockoven 1972). However, because of limits in the treatment methods, because of laws that sent the most difficult patients to the hospitals, and because the hospitals began to fill with the poor and with Irish immigrants, looked on as inferior and untreatable, state hospitals lost public support. Moreover, in the mid 1800s some state hospitals were attacked

1

politically, on the grounds that they incarcerated innocent victims against
their wills (Caplan 1969), attacks somewhat similar to those leveled by Szasz
(1962) in the present day. Because they received meager resources, served the
underclass, and after the first few years discharged relatively few of their patients, state hospitals developed fearsome reputations as places where hopelessly insane, violent people were incarcerated for life (Grob 1966; 1973; Caplan 1969; Rothman 1971; Bockoven 1972). The state hospitals tended to be
isolated from their communities; a parallel system of care also developed,
consisting of proprietary hospitals, some outpatient clinics supported in teaching hospitals, some voluntary social-service agencies, and private practitioners
largely in psychiatry. The private system served the middle class while the
state-hospital system served the underclass (Hollingshead and Redlich 1958).

Because the state-hospital system had no constituency in the middle class,
it was never able to gain substantial public support. State hospitals were frequently overcrowded, had few trained professionals, and in many places the
nonprofessional staff were patronage appointments (Gish 1972) often recruited
from among those willing to work at a poorly paid job with few other rewards.
During World War II, state hospitals were badly neglected. In some places the
hospitals were staffed by vagrants who were given the choice of working there
or going to jail (Brand 1965).

After World War II exposés in the national media of intolerable conditions
in state hospitals (for example, Deutsch 1948; Gorman 1956; Brand 1965)
led to efforts to improve the care of the mentally ill. Contemporary mental-
health theory and research supported the view that large institutions were
inherently bad (for example, Goffman 1961; Joint Commission for Mental
Health and Illness 1961) and that these institutions created as many problems
of chronicity as they cured patients (for example, Scheff 1966; Zusman 1966).
Given this body of professional opinion, the climate of optimism based on
war-time success with the early intensive treatment of soldiers with mental
disorders, and faith that science and technology would produce many more
wonders, national plans were made to reduce the use of large hospitals and to
provide community-based treatment (Foley 1975; Levine 1981).

A series of federal and state court decisions supported the thrust to deinstitutionalization (Stone 1975; Levine 1981). The decisions making it more
difficult to institutionalize patients involuntarily and to hold patients who
were neither dangerous to themselves or to others led to a distinct decline in
the number of patients held involuntarily (Meyer 1974). Moreover, if patients
were institutionalized, they were entitled to a number of personal and legal
rights (See, for example *Wyatt* v. *Stickney* 344 F. Supp. 373, 379–381) including
the right to informed consent when subject to drastic treatment procedures
(for example, lobotomy, electroshock, and aversive reinforcement conditioning),
and the right to consultation with counsel when such treatments are proposed.
Other decisions made it necessary to pay patients wages if they did hospital

work, as patients in many states did [*Souder* v. *Brennan* 367 F. Supp. 808 (D.D.C. 1973); *Wyatt* v. *Stickney*, 344 F. Supp. 373, 379–381]. Equally important, court decisions also required that if patients were treated in the hospital, they be treated in the least restrictive environment [for example, *Lake* v. *Cameron* 364 F. 2d 657 (D.C. Cir. 1966)]. All these factors taken together entered into policy decisions to discharge patients from state hospitals and to provide treatment in the community.

Among the more important but least discussed factors were federal acts (Medicaid and Medicare Amendments to the Social Security Act in 1965, and the Supplemental Security Income amendment in 1972) that provided fiscal incentives for states to reduce their hospital populations. The federal acts provided financial support for the placement of the elderly and the disabled in skilled nursing homes, in health-related facilities, in domiciliaries and in board-and-care homes. The cost of maintaining patients in these facilities is considerably lower than hospital costs. Moreover, since the federal government reimburses states for many of these services, the federal acts made it possible to shift the financial burden from state mental-hygiene budgets to state and local welfare budgets and to the federal budget. Many state mental-health authorities took advantage of these fiscal provisions, through directives to hospitals, or through the exercise of budgetary controls that induced hospital superintendents to reduce hospital populations (U.S. Senate Subcommittee on Long Term Care 1976; Levine 1979).

Deinstitutitionalization and community mental-health programming, initially greeted with enthusiasm, were quickly subject to devastating criticism as journalistic exposés (for example, Witten, Kerr, and Turque 1977; Koenig 1978) and legislative inquiry (for example, U.S. Senate Subcommittee on Long Term Care 1976; Comptroller General of the U.S. 1977) uncovered abuses. Patients were released to nursing homes, to board-and-care homes, or to welfare hotels with little planning and little possibility for after-care. This phenomenon, which might have resulted in the premature deaths of some older, frail patients (Goplerud 1979), came to be called "dumping."

Professional thinking had anticipated the development of a nationwide network of community mental-health centers to provide the outpatient care. Fewer community mental-health centers developed than planners expected, and many of those did not have services appropriate for the chronic clients who were discharged from state institutions (Connery et al. 1968; Lamb and Edelson 1976; Bloom 1977). In the absence of federally funded centers, responsibility for after-care was left to unprepared local communities, on the pious hope that resources would *follow* patients into the community, or to state hospitals that were somehow expected to reorient their missions to provide appropriate care for their former patients, now living outside of the hospital's walls. Although hospital censuses declined drastically, readmission rates either climbed, or remained relatively steady, leading many to speak of the "revolving door"

(President's Commission Task Panel on Nature and Scope of the Problem 1978; Witkin 1979).

Some programs for the after-care of discharged patients were worked out (for example, Lamb, Heath, and Downing 1969; Anthony 1979). The community mental-health literature reported successful attempts to provide appropriate environmental resources and supports for former mental patients to enable them to live in the community (for example, Marx, Test, and Stein 1973; Perry 1979). For the most part, however, progress was slow and piecemeal (see Schulberg and Baker 1975). While some places did initiate partial community-support programs, others reported great resistance to change and little progress. For example, even though the state-hospital system in Alabama was under court order to modify its treatment programs, compliance with the court order was slow, as it was with similar orders in a number of states including New York (Lottman 1976).

Although some critics questioned the thrust of the community mental-health movement from its very beginning (for example, Dunham 1965), and criticism intensified as abuses came to light, despite it all, the most careful professional review we have is that provided by the President's Commission on Mental Health (1978), chaired by Mrs. Rosalynn Carter and Dr. Thomas Bryant. The president's commission held hearings all over the nation and commissioned task forces composed of experts, citizens, and public figures to review each area of mental-health programming. While one may question the politics of the review (see Levine et al. 1981), the commission's report supports the general thrust toward community-based care. Federal policy documents show the Department of Health and Human Services (formerly HEW) is taking the president's commission recommendations very seriously. Community support programs are being developed (Turner, Stone, and TenHoor 1977; HEW Task Force 1979). Since federal policy does not look as if it will change in the foreseeable future, it being rather continuous for nearly thirty years (Levine et al. 1981), Harlem Valley's experience in deinstitutionalizing and in reallocating its resources to community-based programs has something meaningful to say to the community mental-health field for the foreseeable future.

Harlem Valley deinstitutionalized and developed community support programs for its former patients. Its treatment programs in and out of the hospital are not particularly unique. What is unique and worthy of study is the combination of methods used for implementing change within a state institution embedded in a large state bureaucracy, governed by civil-service regulations, limited by a union contract, and constrained further by tradition and all the resistances to change commonly found in organizational settings. It is a truism that efforts at organizational change meet with resistances, often powerful enough to block the change entirely or to subvert its purposes, so that in the end nothing really does change. However, the result was different at Harlem Valley. The institution in 1978 was very different than it was in 1974.

This case report describes how organizational change was accomplished. The study centers on the methods employed by the center's director, Yoosuf A. Haveliwala, M.D. While it is true that Haveliwala is an unusually perceptive and capable executive, he followed a plan and employed recognizable methods. Because the methods are describable, his accomplishment is more than a personal triumph. Rather, he conducted an important experiment in planned organizational change, important because much of what we know about change comes from organizational studies in the private sector. We know very little about the process of planned change in organizations that are part of large governmental bureaucracies.

The changes at Harlem Valley were accomplished without a massive infusion of new resources but by the creative reallocation of existing resources, while still carrying out the everyday routine of a large hospital. Existing resources were not viewed as fixed by job description, position on an organizational chart, or by what had been done in the past. Existing resources were deployed as the tasks required them, supported by an administrative willingness to bend bureaucratic rules in the interests of innovation. The approach to change relied very heavily on data as guides to the progress of change. In contrast to many facilities, program-evaluation data were generated not to produce an annual report for a funding agency but as a management tool used on a day-to-day basis, to monitor change, and to plan future directions. The change effort was abetted by a system of rewards that, surprisingly, were often nonmonetary. Harlem Valley found talented people at all levels in its organization and used administrative discretion to establish conditions that enabled talented and ambitious individuals to exercise their talents creatively.

Harlem Valley's program of change was not without controversy. First, controversy can be expected simply because there usually are good arguments to be made against any program of change, and honest proponents of alternatives feel obligated to assert their positions. Second, the process of change is itself anxiety provoking. Change is not an abstraction. It means job functions change, and along with it there may be losses or gains in status, money, or the amount of work people are required to perform. Relationships also change. Long-time coworkers may be separated, and people must relate to new coworkers and supervisors. Schedules may change. The host of factors, practical and psychological, that must be accommodated lead people to have strong feelings about change. Third, change is implemented by forceful leaders. The leader's style may provoke criticism, or the changed mission may favor some over others. Charismatic leaders elicit strong feelings from their followers, and not everyone's expectation may be met. Fourth, programs were taken out into the community, into a complex of competing governmental and service organizations, and in circumstances in which not all community members welcomed ex-mental patients in their midst.

The relationships with private and public agencies and local government in the communities in which Harlem Valley's support programs were initiated are integral both to the story and to the controversy that developed. The issues arose out of the complicated relationships among state, local, and private mental-health agencies that constituted the task environment within which changes were planned and implemented. If we ever needed convincing that everything really is connected to everything else, instituting change in a complex task environment will provide the evidence.

That change was accomplished is one thing. That it was good is something else. Critics of the deinstitutionalization movement have charged, with good reason, that the effort to empty institutions was in reality an effort to save money at the expense of chronic patients who are not served by remaining in the community in inadequate living quarters, with uncertain nutrition, subject to exploitation, and without supervision or care. We cannot say that we have hard evidence that Harlem Valley's patients were better off in the community than they were in the hospital, or that some patients may not have been released to substandard conditions. It was beyond the scope of this case study to engage in systematic evaluation of the outcomes of deinstitutionalization. However, there appears to be credible evidence in Harlem Valley's own evaluation and follow-up studies and in the reports of its monitoring committees to warrant the judgment that, by and large, its patients were being served as well as the state of the art permits. The arguments in favor of that position will be discussed in the final chapter. For now, we ask the reader to accept it on faith that Harlem Valley's claims that it is serving its patients well can be backed by credible evidence.

If we are to continue in the directions we have undertaken in mental health, as we apparently will, judging from political commitment at a national level to the community mental-health concept, the necessity to provide community supports for the chronic mental patients in our midst is undeniable. The most effective pattern of care is yet to be developed, and if we are to judge from Roosens's (1979) account of community life for chronic mental patients in Geel, Belgium, a community with 700 years of experience in providing community-based care, we need to develop an adequate concept of the limits and potentialities of the good life for the chronically dependent individual, and for his caretaker. But no matter how we conceptualize that goal, to realize it, something will have to change, and someone will have to act to bring about change. This case report describes how planned change was brought about in one institution, in the hopes that the description of the process will serve others who are also working to bring about change in complex, organized settings.

2 Methods and Limitations

This case study was undertaken under contract between the New York School of Psychiatry and Human Services Research and Planning, (HSRP) a private, non-profit consulting firm. Its original purpose was to provide a case study of the organizational change process to be used in inservice training sessions delivered in conjuction with a New York State Office of Mental Health–operated, federally funded, community support system demonstration project. The change process, the strategies and tactics, the problems and the solutions were to be described for that purpose.

This study was not undertaken as an evaluation of the Harlem Valley Psychiatric Center's efforts to develop a comprehensive community support system, nor did we undertake to verify by quantitative study claims of successful community placement and treatment of former mental patients. We believe there is credible evidence to support Harlem Valley's claims that its patients are doing as well as the state of the art permits. We will present the evidence in a section of the final chapter.

The case study is in the tradition of holistic methods as analyzed by Diesing (1971) and described by such writers as Bogdan and Taylor (1975) and Douglas (1976). The method has a close kinship to investigative reporting as described in Bernstein and Woodward (1974), in Anderson and Benjaminson (1976), and as analyzed by Levine (1980).

Although the gathering of data in a holistic study is not systematic in the sense that sampling methods and standardized interviews are not used, it none-theless has its own discipline. Because much of a case study is emergent, the research worker would be overwhelmed without a schema, or a theory, to help make sense of incoming information (Glaser and Strauss 1967). The schema, or theory, is a tentative set of hypotheses, open to modification, or to discarding, if the evidence fails to support the initial view. In this instance, based on preliminary information and on the assumption that leadership would be critical, we developed an outline for the study based on standard concepts of leadership (see Hollander 1978), and upon theories of organization and organizational change (for example, Argyris 1962; 1970; Bennis 1966; Blake and Mouton 1964; Hornstein, Bunker, Burke, Gindes, and Lewicki 1971; Katz and Kahn 1966; Schulberg and Baker 1975).

The case study was guided by the premise that every cultural artifact (for example, programs and organizations) is embedded in a social context consist-ing of people in different roles vis à vis the artifact, with each having different stakes in its continuation or change. In this framework, one attempts to understand the change process as it is perceived from different role perspectives. We worked with a Piagetian definition of objectivity; that is, the recognition that phenomena do indeed appear different when viewed from different perspectives. Thus discrepancies in information from different informants is not treated as unreliability but rather as a reflection of differing organizational positions and perspectives.

While we were interested in the leader's view of the world, it was important to try to pin down those strategies of change that he articulated beforehand. Thus some knowledge of the leader's training and previous experience was important. We wanted to know how the leader perceived the problems and how the leader coped with problems attendant upon change, problems seen from his perspective as resistance to change.

Interviews were semistructured. Levine did most of the interviews himself. John Northman conducted some of them from a general outline of the topics to be covered. The interviewer followed leads that emerged as each interviewee expressed him or herself freely. Usually the interviewer had advance information about the interviewee's role. Questions were tailored to help the informant tell a personal story of the change process. If an informant did not reveal an expected bit of information spontaneously, the interviewer probed for it. Interviewees were asked for specific, anecdotal descriptions and concrete examples of generalizations. The events were collected in concrete form in order to help us appreciate just what was meant by the interviewee. The concrete examples were assumed to stand as "personal myths" in which the essential structure of change was revealed. Sometimes an interviewer would confront an interviewee with a statement made by another informant in order to obtain the second person's view of a particular matter. (We kept confidences and did not identify the source of such statements, nor did we use such statements if they could have been made by only one person.)

Rare factual discrepancies among interviewees often could be reconciled by understanding the comment from the viewpoint of the person who offered it. Most of the time information or events would be described by more than one person. Sometimes, of course, only one individual would have information, and others were not privy to it. We sought documentary evidence in support of statements by examining manuals, official reports, internal reports, committee meeting minutes, and similar records.

About half the interviews were tape recorded with the informant's knowledge and consent. Some requested the interviews be off the record. In other instances, interviews occurred under conditions not conducive to tape recording, or even to taking notes. In those instances, notes were made as soon as possible after the interview or the event. Important information was offered during car rides, in coffee shops, over beers, or at breakfast or dinner.

Although we spent many working days at the Harlem Valley Center, we made but brief visits to the wards themselves. We relied on a recently written report of the Joint Commisssion on Accreditation of Hospitals for information about the quality of inpatient care. We visited only one of the Harlem Valley community clinics, and that on a ceremonial occasion (Mental Health Day) when patients were absent from the clinic. We relied on interviews and documents for information about the outpatient services.

Because some aspects of the Harlem Valley program were controversial, we deliberately sought out people who were known to be critical of Harlem Valley's programs. We also spoke to some ex-employees who had no current interest in Harlem Valley. Some had left to take promotions, and some had left partly because of some conflicts or dissatisfactions. One former employee read a draft of the manuscript and commented on its accuracy from his viewpoint.

Because of our belief in the value of an "adversarial model," and to gain the confidence of those at Harlem Valley, we offered to submit a draft of the manuscript for their review. It was understood that the author would retain editorial control. We welcomed correction of factual errors. Where differences in interpretation arose, we agreed beforehand that we would first attempt to reconcile them. If the differences could not be talked out, then we agreed to include the alternative interpretations in the body of the report. A draft of the manuscript was reviewed by serveral Harlem Valley executives and the director, and their comments were forwarded to us. Some modifications were based on their comments. In general, their comments served to elaborate rather than to change various sections. Although the director indicated that he disagreed with some of the interpretations, he did not request any changes in the manuscript. The feedback was valuable in keeping the report faithful to people's experiences.

We used a knowledgeable other to review our work at several stages, to raise questions about the adequacy of our data, and to suggest areas of inquiry. Dr. Mark Ramsdell, a systems analyst who works as an independent consultant, served in this role several times. Other principals in HSRP (Frank Baker, Douglas Bunker, Drew Hageman, and Raymond G. Hunt) reviewed and commented on the work in its various phases. A colleague, expert in organizations and organizational change, Barbara Bunker, reviewed part of the work in an informal seminar. A number of State University of New York, Buffalo, graduate students also read, commented on, and discussed the monograph in seminars. Mike Ross, then with the New York School of Psychiatry, and now with the New York State Office of Mental Health, followed the work closely. He had his own sources of information about events at Harlem Valley. His comments and leads were helpful in making sure that all perspectives were represented in the case study.

The criticism of knowledgeable reviewers, peers and students, was sought deliberately to introduce this type of control into the case study. We had to be able to be able to answer their questions and criticisms or search for information that would. Their "editorial" review is an example of "adversarial control" in field research and in investigative reporting (Levine 1974, 1980).

We did not document every line by attributing quotations or comments to specific individuals. Although all were fully aware of the purpose of the interviews, some asked that their remarks be considered confidential. Some comments may appear critical of identifiable individuals. To avoid embarassment, the comments are not attributed to the person who made them. The reader will have to trust that statements contained in the body of the report are well documented in interviews, in reports, and in other documents cited here. The list of interviews and the list of documents is included here rather than in a reference section because the listing is important in showing not only the number of interviewees but also their varied roles and perspectives.

Caveat: This study was completed in 1978. Within a few months after it was completed, Dr. Haveliwala left Harlem Valley to take on the directorship of the Creedmoor Psychiatric Center. Wendy Acrish, who was his deputy director, administration, was appointed director. Many of the key employees are still at Harlem Valley, but a few were promoted and left. Harlem Valley is still fighting for its life. It is still one of the psychiatric centers that has been targeted to close down as a hospital and to continue to operate its outpatient facilities only. It may be reorganized as a center for geriatric psychiatric patients. We cannot say how much of its program or its feeling tone survived the change of leadership, nor what changes came about because a new leader, working in a different task environment, defined the mission differently. The events and programs were as we described them through 1978. Although we cannot say the degree to which the methods and organizational spirit did or did not survive the change in leadership because we have not had the opportunity to study the hospital again, the reader should be on notice that the situation may be different in some ways from how it was when we studied Harlem Valley in 1978. This warning is particularly important because the bulk of the monograph is written in the present tense, and the present tense may or may not apply. The present tense is used as a literary device to reflect the living quality of what we observed.

We would like to express our appreciation for the cooperation, and for the candor, which made our task not only exciting but also very pleasant as well. The interviewees and the positions they held at the time are listed below. The reader should examine the list to appreciate the variety of viewpoints that are represented.

Interviews

1. Wendy Acrish, deputy director, administration
2. Arthur Arnold, deputy commissioner, New York State Mental Hygiene Department

3. Rhoda Artus, deputy chief of service, Inpatient Services
4. Marjorie Braren, director, Office of Program Evaluation
5. Roger Christenfeld, consultant in epidemiology
6. Zelda Domashek, West Chester County Mental Health Department
7. Jack Dominguez, unit chief
8. Janice Ek, team leader, Geriatric Service, formerly acting unit chief
9. Ghulam Faruki, formerly deputy director clinical
10. Steven Friedman, West Chester County Mental Health Department
11. Camille Giuditta, director, Volunteer Services
12. Sam Gordon, Board of Visitors, president, Search for Change, Inc.
13. Alifiyah Haveliwala, supervisor, volunteers, outpatient
14. Yoosuf A. Haveliwala, director, Harlem Valley Psychiatric Center
15. Louise Hubbard, executive coordinator
16. Marlene Levin, program evaluation, West Chester County Mental Health Department
17. Rosalie Lichtenstein, nursing-home placement supervisor
18. Don Lund, director, program evaluation, New York State Mental Hygiene Department
19. Esther Malik, Westchester County Mental Health Association
20. William McKenna, formerly personnel officer, Harlem Valley
21. Alvin Mesnikoff, New York Regional Director, New York State Mental Hygiene Department
22. Chung Moon, director, Office of Quality Care
23. Charles Murphy, director, personnel, New York State Mental Hygiene Department
24. George Nash, director, program evaluation, West Chester County Mental Health Department
25. Albert Newman, commissioner of mental hygiene, Dutchess County
26. Burt Pepper, commissioner of mental hygiene, Rockland County
27. Jim Regan, unit chief; director, inservice training
28. Pincus Rosenfeld, formerly unit chief, Southern Westchester Unit
29. Muriel Shepherd, director, Office of Community and Public Relations
30. Dave Sorenson, associate director
31. Jerome Steiner, director, professional training
32. Deena Tannenbaum, Community Support Program
33. Robert Tannenbaum, unit chief
34. Robert Thompson, CSEA-AFCSME local president.
35. Mary Ann Valinski, quality-assurance engineer
36. Martin Von Holden, formerly associate director and unit chief
37. Steve Witte, assistant to deputy director administration
38. Paula Wolfe, formerly director, program evaluation
39. Patricia Wolke, director, mental health, Putnam County
40. William Youngman, Rockland Psychiatric Center

Harlem Valley Reports

Annual Reports, Harlem Valley Psychiatric Center, 1974–1977

Departmental Annual Reports, Harlem Valley Psychiatric Center, 1974–1977

Harlem Valley Quarterly Evaluation Report (1 January 1977–31 March 1977)

1976 HVPC Discharges (One-year follow-up report)

Harlem Valley Psychiatric Center Manuals

Office of Quality Care

Office of Program Evaluation

Quality Assurance Program

Putnam Community Services Policy and Procedures

Placement Service Policy and Procedures

By-laws, Harlem Valley Hospital Medical Staff

Committee Minutes

(Unless otherwise noted, these documents were sampled or scanned.)

Family-care subcommittee

Human Resources Committee

Incident Review Committee

Utilization Review Committee Coordinators

Planning Committee, Office of Planning

Program Review Committee

Program Evaluation Review Committee

Executive Committee (minutes studied carefully for 1974–1975 and thereafter scanned)

Other Reports and Documents

Budget Review and Preparation Memo, 4 February 1975

Proposal, Community Support System, 1977

Letter from John D. Porterfield, to Y.A. Haveliwala, transmitting

Report of Joint Commission on Accreditation of Hospitals, accrediting adult programs for two years, 19 August 1977

Public-relations Handouts and Brochures

HVPC Program Brochures

Dialogue (HVPC newspaper)

Cooperative Industries (May 1978)

Published Works by Harlem Valley Staff

Christenfeld, R., and Haveliwala, Y.A. Patients' views of placement facilities: A participant-observer study. *American Journal of Psychiatry* 135 (1978): 329–332.

Wolfe, P.C., and Haveliwala, Y.A. A model for program evaluation in a unitized setting. *Hospital and Community Psychiatry* 27 (1976): 647–649.

Papers Read at Professional Conferences by Harlem Valley Staff

Acrish W. Address to Association of Mental Health Administrators, September 1977.

Acrish W. Abstract for Program Committee, International Mental Health Administrators, San Diego, Calif., 1977.

Haveliwala, Y.A. Changing a mental hospital. VI World Congress of Psychiatry, 1977.

Unpublished Papers by HVPC Staff or Former Staff

Artus, R. Maintaining quality care despite limited resources.

Bouyea, J.M. Community placement without "dumping" is possible with limited resources.

Dominguez, J. Establishing a rehabilitation program with limited resources.

Ek, J. Effective and extensive outpatient services can develop quickly and effectively with limited resources.

Puglisi, E. A use of family care.

Regan J. Treatment plan implementation with limited staff resources.

Von Holden, M.H. The prospect of limited resources in mental health organizations: Challenge or entropy?

Von Holden, M.H. An analysis of some problems which confront a large, complex service organization as it attempts to adapt to change in its environment in order to survive. (Unpublished paper, undated)

Von Holden, M.H. Management module assignment (Unpublished paper, December 1974)

Von Holden, M.H. We vs. them. (Unpublished paper, March 1975)

Von Holden, M.H. The setting of American public administration module papers (Unpublished, undated).

Environmental forces influencing the southern Westchester Unit of Harlem Valley Psychiatric Center, no. 1.

The social-contextual environment of a rural/suburban community mental health system, no. 2.

Scanning the environment in order to develop appropriate mental health services for eastern Dutchess County, no. 3.

The three most important elements in the task and contextual environment of the Department of Mental Hygiene, no. 4.

Von Holden, M.H. Maximizing available resources by utilizing a "primary therapist model" (Unpublished paper, undated) Unpublished symposium proposal abstracts 1974

Other Publications and Papers

CSEA: To Nowhere and back again. In New York State: The exile of the mentally ill. A CSEA Position Paper (undated).

Fields, S. Unified services. *Innovations,* Winter 1974.

Klein, L.I. Consolidation-realignment of the Department of Mental Hygiene facilities in the Harlem Valley: Economic and sociological impacts. Report prepared for Eastern Dutchess Economic Study Committee, August 1977.

Mesnikoff, A. Organization and staffing. Challenges to theory and practice in community mental health. Proceedings of a Symposium, Fordham University Graduate School of Social Service, 17–18 April 1975.

Mesnikoff, A.M., and Gelber, I. Unified services for an urban population: Response to a fragmented mental health delivery system. Paper presented at American Orthopsychiatric Association Meeting, New York, 31 May 1973.

Mesnikoff, A.M., Haveliwala, Y.A., Berger, M.M., and Cohen, P. South Beach Regional Mental Health System: Serving the gateway communities of New York City. Scientific exhibit. American Psychiatric Association Meeting, Honolulu, Hawaii, May 173.

Mesnikoff, A.M. From restraint to community care: An intersection of historical trends. Paper presented at APA New York District Branches Annual Meeting. 21 November 1969.

3 The Changes

In the summer of 1974 Harlem Valley Psychiatric Center was an institution without much of a future. It was widely believed that the hospital was slated to close, not because its fifty-year-old physical plant was inadequate but because there seemed to be no reason for Harlem Valley's continuation. Located in a rural area of New York State, far from the population centers within its catchment area, its accreditation as a teaching hospital was in danger of revocation. If it did not meet standards set by the Joint Commission on the Accreditation of Hospitals (JCAH), its eligibility for reimbursement for federal and third-party payments would also have been endangered. The hospital had been slow to respond to New York State Mental Hygiene policies and directives and had not accomplished unitization nor any significant reduction in its census until 1974.

On 1 July 1974 the hospital had a total census of 2652 patients, of which 1826 (69 percent) were inpatients with an average hospitalization of 19.5 years, and 826 (31 percent) were outpatients. There were 1000 admissions to the hospital in 1974. The bulk of the 1625.5 full-time equivalent staff were assigned to inpatient care (1535.5, or 94 percent) with only 92 staff (6 percent) assigned to outpatient care. The after-care programs were limited to a few part-time clinics in several districts. Clinical personnel supervised the medication of patients who were released or discharged. The ratio of inpatient clinical staff to hospitalized patients was 1 to 1.8. Of the inpatient staff, 34 percent were in support positions (maintenance, clerical, and so on) and 66 percent were clinical staff. About 80 percent of the clinical staff were paraprofessionals.

With some important and notable exceptions, the then-existing professional staff could be characterized as mediocre. Many of the high-level clinical staff in key roles were dubious about, if not actively opposed to, Department of Mental Hygiene policies. They did not understand or approve unitization, the utilization of team structures, the emphasis on short-term care and early discharge, and especially, the placement of long-term patients in community facilities. After the retirement of its long-time director in 1971, the director was unfilled for long periods. One director retired within 60 days of his appointment, and another director, after having accomplished unitization, a reorganization of the services, left within eighteen months. The director appointed in July 1974 was the third to hold that position since 1971. The impermanence of directors, the transfer of a large number of patients to other facilities, the closing of several buildings, and layoffs all led to the conclusion that the hospital would be phased out.

15

The hospital's budget had been declining for several years, partly as a result of the reduced census (that due largely to transfers to other institutions and deaths within the geriatric population) and partly as a result of Department of Mental Hygiene policy that appeared to be moving toward phasing out the hospital. Some believe it retained its lease on life because local political lobbying prevented its closing. In 1974 its budget was $19,518,842 and the crude, per-patient cost was $8729.36.

In 1974 the hospital had no vigorous recruitment program for professional staff. Its reputation, some say, was as a facility that placed little demand on professional personnel for performance. Its orientation was custodial. Few innovations in treatment programs were being used in most of its services, with one notable exception, to be described later (see chapter 4). Few of the medical staff seemed well versed in the modern use of psychoactive drugs, and treatment plans and medical records were either absent or poor. Aside from an orientation toward keeping patients reasonably clean and involved in routine occupational and recreational programs, there was little sense of mission in the hospital. There seemed to be a symbiotic relationship between staff and patients, in which personnel recognized that care of patients was their reason for being. Personnel enjoyed many fringe benefits. These included housing (many lived in subsidized rental units on the grounds), job security, and a relatively congenial work situation. Personnel prided themselves on their ability to provide a comfortable situation for their patient friends.

There was little in the treatment program to attract well-trained, aggressive, ambitious professional personnel. There was no research and only perfunctory inservice training. Aside from the routine reports required of the institution, there was no evaluation or review of the quality of care. The hospital, however, was a major employer in its geographic area, and many people who were tied to the area found it attractive as the best employment they could find. The hospital, as a reasonably desirable working situation, was able to select competent, responsible, and stable people in many positions, although the clinical leadership in most of its services was not of top-notch calibre.

There was little community involvement. Harlem Valley had a Board of Visitors, with members appointed by the governor, and some volunteer services. Few members of the Board of Visitors were closely identified with Harlem Valley or with many segments of its catchment area. In days past, community leaders used to socialize with the hospital leadership (for example, use of recreational facilities), but there was little involvement in the hospital itself. Political leaders of local communities were concerned about the economic impact of closing the hospital. A few local officials worked in the hospital, and most had neighbors, friends, and relatives who worked there. Local businesses had few contracts with the hospital, but many small businesses benefited from the hospital payroll. Local real-estate values were probably heavily dependent on the existence of the hospital. The volunteer service was not aggressive in seeking out volunteers for the hospital's volunteer program. There was no active public-relations program nor any attempt to present the hospital's merits to the surrounding community.

By 1 July 1977 the hospital's accreditation had been renewed with words of praise by the Joint Commission on Accrediting Hospitals (JCAH) for its progress, for its service program, and for its medical-records package that was cited as a model for other hospitals. Unitization had been accomplished throughout the hospital, and active teams were operating in all units. The mission to reduce the inpatient census by placing patients in appropriate community settings had apparently been accomplished. Unit teams had reduced the hospital's inpatient census more rapidly than most professionals believed possible. Moreover, Harlem Valley could lay claim to having made carefully planned placements, and to having provided follow-up services even when the center's staff boldly placed clients outside of the geographical limits of its designated catchment area.

The hospital census stood at 3068 with 590 *inpatients* (19 percent) and 2478 *outpatients* (81 percent). The hospital had fewer total staff than in 1974. There were only 1207.5 full-time equivalent staff with 181.5 (15 percent) assigned to outpatient services, and 1026 (85 percent) assigned to inpatient care. Of the inpatient staff, 38 percent were classified as support, and 62 percent as clinical. The ratio of inpatient clinical staff to hospitalized patients was now 1 to 0.9.

There are now 30 separate services located in seven communities. These include outpatient clinics offering individual, group and family psychotherapy, and supervision of psychiatric medication; day-care centers, and day hospitals for discharged patients and for geriatric patients; mobile crisis-intervention teams; a housing and sheltered-living program (an independent nonprofit corporation was created to develop housing opportunities for released patients); vocational rehabilitation; sheltered workshops, and work-placement facilities; advocacy services to link clients with community agencies; outreach services including home visits; and efforts to develop cooperative programming with other agencies.

The outpatient services screen referrals for admission to the Harlem Valley Center and provide consultation to families or other agencies to develop alternatives to hospitalization. The center has developed agreements for emergency hospitalization in several communities, and in others a county hospital accepts patients for short-term care. In still others, the center was developing a facility to divert admissions from the formal hospital system. As a result of the availability of community-based services, and Harlem Valley's intention to avoid hospitalization whenever reasonable, admissions in 1977 fell to 350. The implementation of the intention to avoid hospitalization is rigidly monitored through means to be described as follows.

The hospital's total budget for 1977 was $15,184,000. The crude per-patient cost per year had dropped to $4949.50. In other words, both budget and staff have declined while the total number of patients served has increased. Overall (the point is disputed by some line workers, for reasons to be discussed later), the ratio of inpatient staff to in-hospital patients has increased.

Although total staff has decreased, the decline has been heaviest in paraprofessional and support ranks. The number of professional staff has remained relatively constant, and the hospital and its outpatient facilities have been able to attract well-qualified professionals. Where professionals had constituted approximately 20 percent of the clinical staff in 1974, by 1977 professionals constituted almost 28 percent of the clinical staff. The hospital developed a vigorous recruiting program that attracted physicians both to inpatient and outpatient units, and well-qualified, young, ambitious professionals in psychology, social work, and rehabilitation. As Harlem Valley developed a reputation for doing innovative work, and as it developed a reputation for being a facility where merit was recognized (in a variety of ways to be described), it became easier to recruit staff.

Harlem Valley Psychiatric Center now has an extensive in-service educational program directed toward professionals and paraprofessionals. It is accredited by the American Medical Association to offer continuing medical-education credits. It had developed relationships with local community colleges to upgrade the educational level of its nonprofessional employees and has actively encouraged professional employees to seek advanced degrees to qualify them for promotion. Its inservice training programs attempt to relate directly to training needs as these emerge from day-to-day operations. An employee-assistance program to provide counseling to employees was also initiated.

At present eight psychology interns, and twenty students from other disciplines (nursing, occupational therapy, social work, and so on) do field work in the institution. Harlem Valley concluded a training agreement with Cornell University Medical Center to develop a psychiatric-residency and fellowship program in community psychiatry. Through the New York State Department of Mental Hygiene Research Foundation, seminars and conferences bringing nationally known authorities have been supported. These and other training events, including regular Grand Rounds that provide continuing medical-educational credit, are held not only on the hospital grounds but also in community facilities. The training events are open to the professional public. The hospital has developed a media library and video equipment used in supervision and inservice education in each outpatient center.

A key aspect of the Harlem Valley program is its extensive system of monitoring its services. There are a number of evaluative methods in operation. These include a continuing review of the quality of medical records, continuous utilization review, ongoing program review, quality assurance, and program evaluation. Some of the monitoring devices are ongoing reviews that yield quantitative data about the status of patients and the quality of service rendered to patients. Other reviews involve site visits to programs and community facilities in which patients are placed to see that programs are suitable. In addition to the monitoring function, special studies and research projects are suggested by the reviews. There is an epidemiological unit that conducts special studies concerning the needs of populations in given catchment areas for care. Further, there is an active research department that conducts clinical studies of general relevance to the center's mission.

Harlem Valley's system of monitoring its programs is among the most elaborate to be found anywhere. Its approach is important because program evaluation and review data are used systematically in informing a variety of management decisions. Data are used to develop priorities; to identify problems; to suggest directions for solutions; as the basis for new programs; and as the basis for the reallocation of resources within the center. Newly implemented solutions to problems and new and ongoing programs are monitored through the various program-evaluation and review devices.

In fact, much of the social system that is Harlem Valley can be characterized as a series of program efforts monitored by an evaluation procedure to see that programs reach and maintain standards or goals and objectives. One can see such systematic monitoring devices in almost every one of the center's programs. Because the system is characterized by its monitoring devices, with procedures and structures to ensure that corrective action is taken, and these were critical in the change process, they are described in detail in chapter 8.

Community involvement increased strikingly over the four years. As a matter of policy, each outpatient unit developed a community advisory board. Unit chiefs endeavored to select vigorous, active, influential people for their boards. Advisory board members are considered sufficiently important so that regular staff time is allocated to recruiting and working with them. Some who participated on advisory boards were appointed by the governor of New York to the center's Board of Visitors. Members of the Board of Visitors are very actively involved in the center's activities. In addition to the Board of Visitors, a local community advisory body, consisting of influentials (for example, town legislators, county supervisors, and prominent business people) in the communities immediately adjacent to the hospital itself, has been formed to reflect the concerns of the immediately surrounding communities.

Center staff have been encouraged to address their concerns to the state legislators by seeing that their interests are reflected in statements made at legislative hearings and in communications to legislators. The director of the center has been active in the State Hospital Director's Association and has spearheaded lobbying efforts on behalf of state-system programming.

Unit chiefs have themselves participated and encouraged others to participate in community mental-health boards, health-services-administration committees, and in coordinating councils that exist in various communities. Some of this participation in and with community agencies has been facilitated by advisory board members who serve on several service agency boards simultaneously. Professional personnel have also been encouraged to participate and to take leadership roles in local, statewide, and national professional organizations.

Community involvement in voluntary work has increased rapidly over the four-year period. Volunteer hours have increased from 7530 in 1974-1975 to 36,170 in 1976-1977. There is a director for volunteers on inpatient services and another for volunteers for outpatients. Volunteers come from a variety of walks of life, and include students, housewives, retired individuals, and former clients. The two volunteer directors are in constant touch with community agencies to recruit additional volunteers and replacements for those who leave. The volunteer services bring the center's story to a great many people in Harlem Valley's communities

A research department has been productive in that publications emanating from Harlem Valley are appearing in major professional journals. The center has been able to attract some outside funding for research from government agencies and from drug companies. Personnel are encourage to participate in presentations at national and international professional meetings. Harlem Valley has also begun to publish its own journal.

The remarkable transformation has been accomplished during a period of declining resources. The center has followed New York State Mental Hygiene Department policies and budgetary controls, and civil-service and union regulations. Harlem Valley Psychiatric Center had no special relationship to the New York State Mental Hygiene Department to give it favored status. The Harlem Valley Center, under the leadership of its director, is notable for reasons other than that it has reduced its census rapidly; other institutions can show comparable records. More important, the center can claim and document that it has improved care within the institution. In addition, it has developed extensive outpatient and after-care facilities, which have allowed it to reduce readmissions while providing appropriate care for many of the patients it has released into the community.

How was this change brought about? What were the change strategies and tactics? What problems were encountered along the way, and what new problems were introduced by the changes? How were the tensions related to change managed? What favorable factors existed facilitating change? How does the institution continue to identify and manage new challenges? Is any of the methodology replicable, or does it depend on a special blend of leadership and fortuitous circumstances unreplicable elsewhere?

The case study presents a description and analysis of some of the major elements in the process of change. In each instance, we shall try to describe the approach and its merits and the problems that emerged. The case study focuses on those principles and practices that can be described sufficiently to be adapted by others in similar situations.

4 Before the Beginning

Although the appointment of Dr. Yoosuf A. Haveliwala as director of Harlem Valley Psychiatric Center in July of 1974 is a convenient beginning, there is always a "before the beginning" (Sarason 1972). A change process always takes place in relation to an institution's history. In order to appreciate the context of the change effort, it is necessary to describe events preceding his assumption of the directorship, for the change process had begun before he arrived on the scene.

The New York State Mental Hygiene Department is responsible for establishing policies and standards for patient care in institutions located all over New York State. It exercises its supervisory responsibilities through its powers of appointment, through the budgetary process, and through normal bureaucratic regulation of each institution's appointments, expenditures, and practices. The director of a psychiatric center is appointed by the commissioner of mental hygiene after consultation with the center's Board of Visitors. The board consists of a group of citizens, appointed by the governor to provide for community participation in the oversight of each center. Directors are responsible for providing leadership in carrying out the center's therapeutic purposes, in carrying out New York State Mental Hygiene policies, and in maintaining standards. Although the institutions are part of a larger system, by virtue of statute, regulations, traditions, distance from Albany, and historically determined separation from their communities, directors have a great deal of autonomy in carrying out their responsibilities.

Harlem Valley Psychiatric Center, located in rural Wingdale, New York, in Dutchess County about 75 miles north of New York City, was built in 1924 as a correctional facility. With overcrowding of New York City mental-health facilities, it was converted to a state mental hospital in 1925. At the peak of its census, it housed nearly 6000 patients, many of whom came from New York City and from Westchester County, 60 miles south of the hospital. Although located in eastern Dutchess County, that area is not included within the hospital's formally designated catchment area.

By 1974 its census was less than half of what it was at its peak. Beginning about 1965 New York State Mental Hygiene Department policies, financial benefits to the states in federal programs (Medicare, Medicaid, Title XIX, and Title XX funds), professional thinking about the problems of large institutions, and the developing community mental-health-centers movement led to efforts to place patients in facilities other than mental hospitals. A series of federal-court decisions strongly influenced mental-hospital practices. These decisions asserted that individuals could be involuntarily confined to mental institutions only if they were dangerous to themselves or others; that if confined, they were entitled to be treated in the least restrictive alternative; and that patient labor that was nontherapeutic had to be paid at minimum wages. Older patients were transferred to nursing homes and similar facilities. Admission to mental hospitals of older patients was more rigidly regulated. At Harlem Valley prior to 1973 the decline in census was less attributable to efforts to deinstitutionalize than to the death rate among elderly hospital patients.

With the decline in census in hospitals all over the state, Harlem Valley's future existence was threatened since its remaining polulation could well be absorbed by other hospitals that now had space. In fact, prior to 1973 the decline in its census was partly the result of the transfer of several hundred patients to other state institutions.

People in the immediate vicinity depended heavily on Harlem Valley for employment. Local businesses and the local housing market benefited from people and money brought into the area by Harlem Valley. The prospects of its closing presented a severe economic threat to the whole area. The economic threat made the prospect of deinstitutionalization unpalatable to many employees. Among some employees, however, the idea that one might save the hospital became a motivating force in favor of innovation.

Until 1973 the hospital had given lip service to the idea of unitizing. It changed the name of some of its services. Basically, however, it was organized according to standard classifications. It had acute and chronic services, both male and female, a medical-surgical service, and geriatric wards. Its program was custodial in orientation. Physicians were in charge of all the units. The hospital operated within a medical model not only in its choice of physicians as leaders of units but also in its goal of attempting to cure illness before releasing patients. Patients received medications. There were some work and recreational programs but little intensive effort to return patients to the community. Many staff members had friendly and familiar relations with long-term patients. Although a preaccreditation survey did turn up difficulties inpatient care (for example, the use of restraints; the cleanliness of some areas of the hospital), for the most part patients were treated kindly. They were fed regularly, kept clean, and were not often subject to serious abuse. The nursing and the paraprofessional staff, drawn from the immediate area, were stable family people whose friends and relatives worked in the institution. Many of their fathers and mothers had worked there before them, and there was a tradition of kindly care. The physical plant was in good condition.

In 1973 Dr. Anthony Primelo arrived as director, after the director preceeding him stayed but sixty days. Dr. Primelo brought with him psychologist Martin Von Holden who was made chief of the then-designated metro unit. Von Holden was the only nonmedical unit chief in the hospital, and his appointment raised eyebrows among the medical staff. Dr. Primelo undertook to reorganize the hospital according to geographic units, in keeping with Mental Hygiene Department policy, and in preparation for discharging and releasing patients back to their communities of origin.

The reorganization took place rapidly. His staff determined patients' original places of residence, assigned them to the appropriate geographic unit, and assigned the geographic units to appropriate hospital buildings. Reassignment of personnel and of patients was accomplished in a single day. All patients were color-coded according to the services they were to be housed in. They were gathered outdoors. Personnel from each newly formed unit led the patients to their new quarters.

This reorganization was accomplished swiftly and smoothly. Dr. Primelo was assisted in the venture by Von Holden, and an experienced nurse, Rhoda Artus, who knew Harlem Valley, and was respected by the staff. The architects of reorganization, familiar with the hospital's culture, took one important step to minimize resistance to the changes on the part of staff. Staff were consulted about reassignment beforehand. It became clear that shift changes were most difficult for many people (for example, second jobs and mothers who wished to work the same shift). Based on the intitial survey, wishes of staff were respected. Although individuals were assigned to new services, no one was required to change shifts.

Reorganization was accomplished but not much else. The hospital went its own way, except in the one service led by Martin Von Holden. Von Holden had charge of metro, a unit oriented toward New York City. An energetic young man, with remarkable ability to motivate others, Von Holden proceeded to organize his service into true teams. He was fortunate in that he had several strong team leaders in his group, social workers Jack Dominguez and Jacqueline Bouyea, nurse Elsie Puglisi, and psychologist Jim Regan. The five of them working together discharged patients rapidly into the New York City area. Later they were joined by Robert Tannenbaum who had worked with another of the units.

They used hospital personnel to develop day-care and visiting programs in some of the neighborhoods where their discharged patients lived. They sent mobile teams on a daily basis (a drive of more than two hours) to the Rockaways, where boarding homes and old hotels provided residences for the released patients. Although this tactic led to charges of "dumping" in another hospital's catchment area, Von Holden was able to show that however difficult it was, he and his staff were following their patients. (In these days some Harlem Valley patients were returned to other areas of New York City, the Bronx, Brooklyn, Manhattan, and Staten Island. Records indicate that about 60 patients were placed outside of the Rockaways. It is not clear that all these patients were followed on a daily basis.) Eventually the conflict was resolved when the other hospital took responsibility for the patients. However, the principle of using mobile teams of inpatient workers to service-released patients on an outpatient basis was established and tested during this early experience.

Von Holden and his group continued to be rate busters in the sense that they outstripped the other units and showed by their efforts that deinstitutionalization without dumping could be accomplished. It was not only deinstitutionalization that was tested. Von Holden had introduced a team structure and also the idea of following patients into the community. He monitored patient progress so that questons about each one's status could be answered. Later as his unit's census was declining, Von Holden realized that he would be rewarding his staff by putting them out of jobs. He then requested that Dr. Primelo assign another catchment area to him so that he could have inpatient and outpatient responsibilities. After some negotiation, he received a portion of Westchester County from another unit chief, gaining additional patients and additional staff.

The transfer of a portion of a catchment area, additional responsibility, and additional staff to a unit chief who had accomplished more than others established a precedent for later action in the center. It also created tension for other personnel. At this point Dr. Primelo felt that he had moved the hospital along toward reorganization and deinstitutionalization, and for personal reasons, decided to leave after having served for about eighteen months.

Dr. Yoosuf Haveliwala, then forty-four years old, is among the first generation of state psychiatric center directors formally trained in the concepts and practices of community psychiatry (See Bindman and Spiegel 1969; Golann and Eisdorfer 1972; Kiev 1969; Lamb, Heath, and Downing 1969). Born in India, he was educated at Bombay University receiving his medical degree in 1957. He did his psychiatric residency at the Buffalo Psychiatric Center, and the Meyer Memorial Hospital, clinical centers affiliated with the SUNY Buffalo Department of Psychiatry. The Division of Community Psychiatry, at that time under the direction of Dr. Jack Zusman, also offered a program in mental-health administration that emphasized modern management techniques, service evaluation, and a public-health orientation. Dr. Haveliwala eventually completed an Master of Public Health degree at SUNY Buffalo. In reflecting on the background that influenced his current thinking, he commented that he absorbed the public-health philosophy, and the combination of the scientific, the evaluative, and the managerial from his Buffalo teachers.

Dr. Haveliwala also functioned as a staff member of the Buffalo Psychiatric Center during its deinstitutionalization efforts. He had the opportunity there to observe problems in deinstitutionalizing. He undoubtedly received some education in state-county tensions since these existed as they still do in most New York communities. While at Buffalo he undertook to develop a day-care program cooperatively with the Meyer Hospital, a county facility, using the principle of shared staffing.

In 1972 he moved to the South Beach Psychiatric Center as deputy director, clinical. South Beach was a brand new showcase facility, under the direction of

Dr. Alvin Mesnikoff. Dr. Mesnikoff had a set of concepts that guided his development of the community-oriented program at South Beach (see unpublished papers by Mesnikoff cited in chapter 2). He believed that the leadership must have clear vision, firm purpose, an independent stance, and the will to pursue purpose in the face of obstacles. He believed that evaluation and feedback were necessary to monitor programs and keep them on target.

He employed a concept he called "creative tension," in which competition among units was encouraged to generate the energy for problem solving. (This concept has its problems since competition among units creates tensions among units that require management. In some situations creative tension can lead to deep enmities among personnel in different groups.) Mesnikoff also believed in participatory management and cooperation across organizational lines. He used interdisciplinary committees to foster these ends. He further believed that good people select good people, so he carefully selected his key personnel and then gave them reasonable autonomy to be creative and energetic (see McGregor 1960; Likert 1961).

In his view, State Mental Hygiene Department and civil-service regulations were not meant as obstacles to implementing public policy or the delivery of services. He believed regulations should be interpreted and if necessary bent to support service delivery. Most important, he felt that community-based programs should be firmly embedded in their communities. Moreover, if they were to generate community and political support for their continuation and development, programs must serve mutual need.

While Dr. Haveliwala fashioned his own approach, there are some important similarities in the principles employed in South Beach and Harlem Valley. It is important to note these because they suggest that the basic elements and principles of an approach are teachable and applicable to a new situation. While any approach will necessarily have to be adapted to the specifics of a situation and will be molded by the social context as well as the personality of the leader, certain consistencies can be noted. For example, many of Dr. Haveliwala's staff credit him with great foresight in anticipating problems as consequences of given actions. One could entertain the hypothesis that his foresight is based less on mysterious intuition than it is on previous experience in implementing similar practices in similar settings. Change agentry may well be a teachable skill, requiring experience in a related setting.

At any rate, when Dr. Haveliwala arrived at Harlem Valley from South Beach, he had been educated in concepts of community psychiatry; was experienced in their implementation; had training and experience in modern management; and he had a public-health outlook. We turn now to see how he, his executives, and his staff put experience and concepts to work introducing change in Harlem Valley.

5 The Change Process

Social organizations persist through time and through changes in their environments because they have structures that contribute to their continuation. If they did not have such structures, their very survival as stable organizations would be questionable. It follows that any change will be difficult simply because organizational continuity requires that the organizations's structural features be relatively resistant to change. It is because successful, planned change is so difficult that we have had a social-science literature and a technology develop around this very question (Argyris 1962; Bennis, Benne, and Chin 1961; Bennis 1966; Hornstein, Bunker, Burke, Gindes, and Lewicki 1971; Sarason 1971).

The problems of change are particularly complex in bureaucratically organized facilities in which employee activities are defined by civil-service regulations, and by union agreements and in which the hire-fire power of the leadership is constrained. Moreover, human-service agencies have their own special characteristics (Demone and Harshbarger 1974; Hasenfeld and English 1975) that complicate the process of planned change. In particular, their exchanges with their environments, to use system terms (Schulberg and Baker 1975), are indirect. Human-service agencies do not usually have clear indices of their productivity, and because they obtain their budgets from legislative action rather than from direct exchanges of resources with organizations or individuals in their task environments, they have less immediate need to be responsive to variations in the task environment.

The process of planning and implementing change is generally difficult, but it is more complex in bureaucratically organized, civil-service-regulated human-service organizations. As Graziano (1969) observed, although human-service organizations are sensistive to the necessity for change, too often the motto seems to be "Innovation without Change." While there are theories of planned organizational change, much of the literature is written from the perspective of external change agents. Frequently these are consultants who have been called in to assist an organization to solve some ongoing problem. A great deal of the organizational change literature is based on experience in private industry. Much less has been written about organizational change from the point of view of formal leaders, and still less from formal leaders functioning within human-service agencies such as psychiatric centers. In approaching the problem of change, Haveliwala would find little direct guidance in the formal literature on organizations or organizational change.

Hornstein, Bunker et al. (1971) have classified change tactics into a number of categories. The first is termed an individual approach. This tactic assumes that organizational difficulties arise from individual failure. The key individuals may not possess the technical skills, they may not communicate well, they may hold attitudes dysfunctional for change, or their personalities may not be suited to the tasks facing them. The individual approach seeks to change individuals through training, personal counseling, or more often through sensitivity or T-groups. As we shall see, Haveliwala eschewed this approach in favor of changing the job responsibilities of those in key positions who were unable to assist in the effort to meet organizational goals, and in favor of selecting new people who were more attuned to the new organizational goals and demands. More important, he restructured the rules for taking on leadership responsibility so that he was able to call on those with the necessary skills and energy to perform a job, independently of rank or formal title.

A second approach has been termed the "technostructural." In this approach, jobs are redesigned so that both human needs and task requirements are considered. Job redesign may include changes in the size of a group performing a task, changes in its composition, changes in physical arrangements, or changes in the tasks that are performed. Sometimes larger organizational features are redesigned to facilitate interdepartmental cooperation and to reduce competition among groups.

Haveliwala did encourage some technostructural changes. These included his support for the unit and team structure that had been introduced by the previous director. Unit chiefs and team leaders also restructured their groups to facilitate cooperation and cohesivenesss in carrying through plans that were developed. Individuals were held accountable for performance but were given great latitude in carrying out their jobs. Haveliwala also restructured the institution's executive committee, changing the size of that body, its composition, its tasks and responsibilities, and its mode of functioning. The frequent organizational changes that will be described are further examples of technostructural changes designed to cope with specific organizational problems.

A third approach to organizational change has been termed "data based." In a data-based approach, the change agent collects information appropriate to organizational issues and attempts to create organizational structures that will employ the information in the change process. One important form of such data-based tactics is evaluation research aimed at demonstrating that any given effort is moving toward meeting its goals. Information that is fed back into the organizational structure to guide it requires a format for using and interpreting the data. Haveliwala made extensive use of such a data-based strategy in promoting change at Harlem Valley. The extensive monitoring and feedback systems that were put into place and used reflect the key role that data-based tactics played in the overall change effort. We shall describe these in some detail in this chapter.

Hornstein et al. (1971) discuss organization-development tactics as a fourth method for producing organizational change. Organizational development aims to create a culture within the organization supportive of continuous review and regulation of its state of functioning. In contrast to episodic and temporary interventions, organizational development aims to develop structures that will support continuous, flexible problem solving. Haveliwala's aim to install a "spirit of inquiry" (chapter 8) seems consistent with the organizational-development aim to create a culture supportive of continuous, flexible problem solving. Moreover, the creation of departments and divisions to develop data, and the creation of executive bodies, and norms within those executive bodies for using data to guide change, is also consistent with organization development aims. Further, Haveliwala's willingness to change the organizational structure as new problems emerge may also be viewed as an important contribution toward creating the desired organizational culture.

Although we can identify components of a change effort and can interpret them in relation to familiar concepts in the organizational literature, each situation is different. Approaches to change must be adapted to the particular details and to the particular factors of any given situation. In what follows, we shall be presenting a description of the change effort as we have been able to reconstruct it from an examination of documents and from interviews with participants. The real world does not come packaged in units and in events that match our analytic categories. In reality, everything is significant of everything else. In what follows, we will describe the moves and phases in change. The reader will have the burden of identifying components in the complex events.

Opening Moves

Although Haveliwala knew Harlem Valley might close, he was unconcerned about a long-term job for himself. He took the position because he wanted to do the things he wanted to do. Interestingly, the Board of Visitors did not really know what he wanted to do when they agreed to his appointment. They asked only if he was going to stay. He had little discussion with them or with the New York State Mental Hygiene Department about his philosophy or his intentions for the hospital. He had no special mandate from either the Board of Visitors or the state, nor any assurance of special resources as an incentive to take the position. He did know there were some strong young staff members at Harlem Valley.

Staff also did not know if he was going to stay or what he was going to do. Having just experienced some important changes, many were uneasy about what was to come next. Some of the professional staff were hoping for a return to the custodial orientation of the recent past. Others were more dubious. The rumor mill had it that Dr. Haveliwala was there to empty out Harlem Valley just as he had done at Buffalo, a psychiatric center that had reduced its patient census rapidly while he was a member of its staff.

On arrival at Harlem Valley, he had a very clear idea of just what he wanted to do. He had a program and some change strategies in mind. One of the first steps he took was to consult briefly with Martin Von Holden, to share some of his plans with him and to obtain an agreement from Von Holden to stay on. Von Holden then left for a vacation. Haveliwala asserted his authority swiftly and dramatically at the first formal meeting with his executive committee, on 9 July 1974. He disclosed his intentions: patients would continue to be placed in the community; each released patient would be provided with a placement appropriate to the patient's needs; and excellent care would be provided to all patients.

His executive committee included some fifty people. The first order of business was his announcement that the presently constituted executive committee (EC) was too large to function as a deliberative and a decision-making body. He therefore was going to establish a smaller body, able to thoroughly discuss institutional problems. Representatives on the new EC would be responsible for obtaining and presenting ideas and information from employees, from patients, and from community members. They would also be responsible for communicating all decisions reached by the EC to all employees and patients. He said he would also form a program committee responsible for long-term planning, for establishing organizational priorities, for reviewing present plans and programs, and recommending changes.

During the initial meeting, the director spoke briefly to each person, asking about each one's role in the hospital. He then presented a list of fourteen people to comprise the new EC. These included the deputy director, clinical; the deputy director, administration; the personnel officer; the business officer; the plant superintendent; the director of education and training; the chief occupational therapist; the director of communications; the five unit chiefs including Von Holden; and one team leader. After some discussion with the group, he agreed to add the chief of nursing, a representative of the four chaplains, and the director of volunteer services. Haveliwala emphasized his intention to strengthen the roles of the units in the decision-making process as opposed to the professional disciplines. After further discussion, during which some additional suggestions were rejected, he thanked the larger group and requested that the newly reconstituted EC meet that same morning.

At 11:00 that same morning, the new EC met. It broke for lunch, and continued to meet the rest of the afternoon. A still smaller program committee was formed, and a time set aside for its meeting. Then Haveliwala set forth guidelines under which the new EC would meet:

1. Decisions would not be made in secret but would be fully aired in the EC meetings.
2. The EC was advisory to the director. While most decisions would be reached by concensus, he reserved the right to make the final decision with which

others might disagree. However, once a decision was reached, he expected full commitment by all to those decisions, and he expected the decisions to be carried out with enthusiasm.

3.   He also emphasized that the primary responsibility of all employees was to the director. If there was any discrepancy between New York State Mental Hygiene Department policies and Harlem Valley practices, Dr. Haveliwala should be advised of the problem, and he would decide what to do.

Establishing his authority by word and by deed, he began to establish norms for the EC's functioning, and he initiated new programs. Most of the lines of development of subsequent programs were foreshadowed in statements made and in actions taken in the first EC meeting.

In sum, the director stated that the major priority of the center was to accomplish a rapid reduction of the inpatient census. However, he emphasized that each patient should be provided with an appropriate community placement and appropriate after-care. The idea that each patient should be placed in an environment therapeutic for that patient and that no patient be discharged or placed in the community without careful planning and follow-up was reiterated several times during the meeting.

The director's emphasis on the quality of care is important to note, for some staff viewed him as pressing only for the rapid discharge of patients. In fact, in his role as leader, he continually pressed for rapid discharge. However, his emphasis on the quality of care is repeated throughout published documents and policy and procedure manuals. Almost every one begins with a preamble stating an intention to provide the highest quality of care, humane care, or loving care. The words differ because each unit developed its own manuals, but the concept permeates all documents. Moreover, there are a number of mechanisms (review committees; formal monitoring devices) designed to assure that humane care of high quality is provided. The organization committed a portion of its resources to such activities. The emphasis on quality of care is an important antidote to the tendency to simply dump patients in the name of deinstitutionalization.

The director anticipated important objections to the objective of reducing the institutional population. By reducing the inpatient population rapidly, the hospital staff would in the long run have better staffing ratios. The staff would be able to provide better care for the remaining patients. Further, the hospital's value to the community would be enhanced by developing additional catchment areas, and new programs for underserved populations (for example, alcoholics, adolescents, and mentally retarded). A deinstitutionalization program accompanied by the development of community-based services would preserve rather than lose jobs. While he committed himself to prevent the loss of jobs, he repeated his determination to reduce the inpatient census. He stated that Harlem Valley employees would lose their jobs only because of incompetence or resistance to the hospital's new directions and programs.

In line with the objective of reducing the inpatient census, each unit chief was directed to submit a plan for ward consolidation. Those plans were to be ready for presentation at the EC meeting within the next few weeks, each unit to be presenting in turn.

He expected still more. Each unit was to develop a therapeutic milieu to provide a more stimulating and humanized environment in the hospital. Each unit was to strive to develop a full range of community-based services, either by using hospital resources or by negotiating for services with existing community agencies. In order to see that objectives were met, he announced his intention to develop an accountability system throughout the center. (In fact, one of the first new employees he hired was Paula Wolfe who had developed a program-evaluation system at South Beach. The accountability system is critical in the change process and will be described in some detail in chapter 8).

The minutes of the first EC meeting record that a number of actions were started (for example, a committee to start discussion with an association of owners of proprietary homes and discussion with the community college to develop educational programs for employees). Dr. Haveliwala announced the appointment of five new physicians. He also said he wanted to appoint an executive coordinator and would prefer promoting someone from within the organization.

At this time Martin Von Holden was the only nonmedical unit chief. He had started to place patients in the community under the previous director. Von Holden had helped create the unit system, and he had formed interdisciplinary teams led by other than medically trained personnel. In this first meeting Haveliwala stated that the interdisciplinary structure would be continued and expanded. He said that he stood behind the previous reorganization. He fully supported the departure from a departmentally dominated organization and the departure from the model of medical-administrative leadership. Later his support of an interdisciplinary structure proved critical. He was able to find competent managers and to appoint people to leadership and supervisory positions irrespective of their disciplinary training. This step increased the number of talented people he could call on.

In this and subsequent meetings, he showed he was serious about change. In a subsequent EC meeting, he instructed his personnel officer to obtain and distribute guidelines for private practice by staff professionals. While there was no evidence that anyone was abusing those privileges, he indicated his intention to keep staff within the state's rules. He also engaged in a discussion of the degree of use of housekeeping personnel to serve staff living quarters on the grounds. (The amount of staff used for this function was questionable, especially in light of a preaccreditation survey that found a number of deficiencies in housekeeping on the wards.) He initiated a discussion of policy toward staff who did not adequately maintain their quarters. Private practice, housekeeping for staff quarters, and the cleanliness of staff quarters must be sensitive issues within the small world of the rural hospital. Undoubtedly, everyone knew who was being discussed even though the minutes record no names. In large and small ways, he signaled his intention to carry out his program and his willingness to take on tough problems.

That first meeting of the newly formed EC made it absolutely clear there was no going back. If anyone had doubts or hopes before, there were few afterwards. It was clear the hospital was going to reduce its census rapidly. The interdisciplinary-team structure using nonmedically trained personnel in leadership positions was to be continued and strengthened. Moreover, the new director was intent on introducing accountability into the system. Shortly after the first meeting, the deputy director, clinical, and all the physician unit chiefs resigned, setting the stage for further developments. (Haveliwala apparently had faith in his ability to recruit physicians. He was not intimidated by the threat of physicians' leaving. His staff, particularly after Ghulam Faruki, M.D., was appointed deputy director, clinical, conducted a vigorous recruitment campaign.)

In most treatises on change agentry, the change agent is urged to take time to assess the particular situation and to become acquainted with the actors before taking action. In this instance Haveliwala acted quickly and decisively. We do not know how much advance information he had about the institution. He did have the opportunity to consult with Von Holden before he assumed his duties as director. It is also true that the state mental-hygiene system is a closed world in which the principal actors know each other, if not personally then by reputation. Moreover, in that small world, there is an active grapevine. Personnel within the system have some idea about the character of each institution. Probably the most important factors were his understanding of the nature of a state psychiatric center from his experience within the system and his appreciation of the statutory and regulatory authority and responsibilities of a facility director. He had functioned as a deputy director under a vigorous director at South Beach, and he was on staff when the Buffalo Psychiatric Center was also led by very active administrators. He unquestionably knew what he could do from a legal viewpoint. He also knew that staff always felt uncertainty with the coming of a new leader especially since there had already been some recent changes that had shaken the staff's complacency. In acting decisively at the beginning, he was exercising leadership in a condition of uncertainty, a condition under which a strong leader can usually make his or her will prevail.

Developing the Position

The resignation of the deputy director, clinical, and the unit chiefs simplified some of the problems of change since it made it possible to move people sympathetic to the new program into positions of responsibility. Martin Von Holden was appointed *acting* deputy director, clinical, and several of the team leaders who supported his efforts to place patients in the community became *acting* unit chiefs in a new reorganization. (Haveliwala made extensive use of acting titles. He also created titles that do not exist in the civil-service structure to accommodate new functions and to place the people he wanted into responsible positions independently of their paper credentials. The advantages and problems in this approach will be discussed in the section on nonfinancial incentives, to follow.) These individuals, social workers Jack Dominguez and Robert Tannenbaum, and psychologist Jim Regan were to prove to be key people who worked closely with Haveliwala in executive roles to carry out a variety of responsibilities. He also appointed Louise Hubbard (she had been an administrative assistant) executive coordinator. Her appointment was important since she had preceded Haveliwala to the hospital and had friendly and mutually respectful relationships with many of the key staff. Ms. Hubbard became an important link between Dr. Haveliwala and the staff.

By August a further reorganization had taken place. The metro unit that had been under Von Holden was discontinued. The Westchester County unit was broken into three services, Northern, Central, and Southern Weschester, each under an acting unit chief with both inpatient and outpatient responsibilities. In mid-September of that first year, psychologist Paula Wolfe joined the staff as program evaluator. She was added to the EC. In November of 1974, Ghulam Faruki, a psychiatrist who was the director's friend and confidante, came to the center as deputy director, clinical. His assignment was to develop the inpatient clinical program to ensure that the hospital received full accreditation.

Using the principle that good people select good people, he appointed committees to search for new professional personnel sympathetic to the center's program. His unit chiefs approved the selection of new people, but he reserved final authority for himself. The acting unit chiefs were encouraged to select team leaders and to assign personnel to duties using the same principle of selecting talented, highly motivated people independently of formal status and paper credentials.

When Faruki took over as deputy director, clinical, Von Holden was appointed associate director (a nonexistant title). He and Faruki divided responsibilities. Most of the unit chiefs reported through Von Holden, and the geriatric and medical and surgical chiefs reported through Faruki. Haveliwala used his authority to delegate responsibilities and to specify reporting relationships. It did not matter that some supervisors and administrators had lower civil-service classifications (and pay) than those they supervised. (Civil-service regulations and provisions of the union contract prohibit directors from *ordering* employees to work outside of their job descriptions. However, if employees *volunteer,* they can fulfill new roles indefinitely. Wendy Acrish then-personnel officer, later deputy director, administration, and still later Haveliwala's successor as director, was a key person in helping to deal with civil-service and union constraints.)

The selection of personnel generally sympathetic to the hospital's program made change easier, but that is far from the whole answer. Staff embarked on new ventures for which few had any real preparation. (Actually, all the key staff had had some experience in similar programs elsewhere. It is safe to say that they had learned by making some of their errors elsewhere.) Moreover, the director's strategy required a rapid reduction of the inpatient census in order to free personnel for duties in outpatient settings. The demand for rapid action put further pressure on the executive staff, and they in turn had to deal with their staffs. Even though most of those in leadership positions around whom resistance to the change could have been organized left, many of the remaining staff had their doubts about the wisdom and desirability about the hospital's new thrust. It was necessary to work closely with all staff to ensure that the hospital's program would be carried out.

6 Strategies for Change

The terms "strategies" and "tactics" derive from military use. Strategy is the science and art of design to meet an enemy in combat under advantageous conditions. Tactic is defined as the science and art of disposing or maneuvering troops in action, or more generally any adroit device for accomplishing an end. While changing a mental hospital may not be the equivalent of going into battle (after all, there should be no enemy), nonetheless, change requires a design that includes certain objectives, and it includes plans for adroit devices to accomplish defined ends. It is probably true that change for its own sake characterizes efforts in many institutions. When a change is proposed, one must always ask, "What is the problem for which the proposed change is a solution?"

A change agent is at a considerable advantage when clear goals and objectives can be specified. While the choice of goals and objectives reflects value-based decisions, the choice of strategies and tactics to achieve goals can be evaluated by whether or not one is making progress toward clearly defined goals. A feedback system cannot operate to keep a system on target if there is no clearly specified target (Von Bertallanfy 1968).

In this instance New York State policy to support community-based treatment and rehabilitative efforts, as expressed in the current mental-hygiene law (Mental Hygiene Laws, Chapter 251, as amended to 14 April 1978), provided the goals and the targets. In this instance there was a fortunate congruence between Haveliwala's professional commitment to modern community mental-health practice and state policy. His change efforts reflected his own professional views and were directed toward implementing state policy.

Even with a target, there is still the problem of finding new resources, or reallocating old ones to meet new objectives. Resources are of two kinds: human and material. Both exist in limited quantity, and one must assume that both are in use in maintaining the organization's existing functions. The simplest form of change is to add on. No one loses when additional resources can be brought to bear, and existing operations can continue to function. However, when resources have to be reallocated, the situation is far more complex. If ongoing functions have to be maintained with reduced resources, then the reduced resources must be used more efficiently in order to accomplish the job. Usually the more efficient use of resources means that the people who do the job have to put in more time or more effort. While it may be true as a theoretical proposition that most organizations tolerate considerable waste and inefficiency, the bald statement of that proposition fails to recognize that it is a criticism of the effectiveness of the workers involved.

Most people do not take criticism of their work lightly. Moreover, many people enjoy the work they do, and others have adapted to it. If they have given up or never had ambitions for promotion, or if they find their positions less than fully challenging, then workers obtain satisfaction in their relationships with their colleagues, or they organize their jobs so that their energies are devoted to outside interests (Kanter 1977). A change may well interfere with job functioning, with ongoing social relationships that provide job satisfactions, or with aspects of one's overall life style.

Change is also challenging. While one's work may become routine, still one can accomplish daily ends and master the familiar problems. A worker takes pride in the skills he or she is exercising and in coping with the job's trials and tribulations. The opportunity for new experiences is exciting to some, but to most who have learned to learn under conditions that threaten self-esteem, the challenge for new learning may reawaken old psychic wounds. After all, for many the experience of learning was as a dependent child, subject to adult criticism and punishment, and vulnerable to failure in competition (Henry 1963). To be asked to take on new tasks may well provoke anxiety.

The call to change is also a criticism of what exists. In the instance of a human-service organization such as a hospital, in which the staff take pride in providing care for other human beings, it is indeed demoralizing to be told implicitly, if not explicitly, that what one has been doing is not helpful but may indeed be harmful. A professionally trained person also commits a great deal of his or her lifetime to achieving professional status. Professionally trained staff are taught to believe that the methods they employ are based on scientific principle, and it is the essence of professionalism to make one's own decisions about the type of service that will be in the client's best interests. Professionals who are committed to one form of practice, who take pride in the exercise of professional skills, and who indeed see their economic value and social position as deriving from the exercise of professional skills, cannot be expected to welcome criticism of their practices.

A state mental hospital is a complex society involving several thousand people, as many as live in small towns. An inpatient population must be served twenty-four hours a day, seven days a week. The population must be housed, fed, dressed, cleaned, occupied, recreated, medicated, and moved from one location to another to fulfill these various functions. In addition to the staff's providing direct patient care, the hospital requires a maintenance staff to keep the physical plant going. It requires a clerical staff to keep the smooth flow of communications and orders going and to keep the necessary records. It also requires a business staff to see that financial accounts are in order and that funds are spent appropriately. It further requires an administrative staff to oversee the various operations and to ensure their coordination. In theory each person has a necessary job to do, and in theory the jobs are interrelated. If some of the jobs do not get done, eventually patient care, the institution's reason for being, will suffer.

Although the language of systems theory is prone to identify patients as inert materials that are processed, patients in a hospital are far from inert. Patients are active, willful human beings pursuing their own ends, even when these ends make little sense from the point of view of rational society (Braginsky, Braginsky, and Ring 1969). Patients in a hospital adapt to its routines, and make a life within it (Goffman 1961). Part of that life includes relationships with familiar personnel. While life in a hospital filled with chronic patients may seem highly routinized, with the routine broken by stochastically predictable, if inexplicable, episodes of break with routine, its stability depends on a dynamic equilibrium. A change in activities or in personnel interferes with the dynamic equilibrium and must create new demands for adaptation for both patients and personnel. Any change effort must reckon with the consequences for patient activity and patient care.

A psychiatric center, even an isolated one, does not function separately from the larger environment. For one, it accepts some patients from the community and it releases others back to the community. For another, it functions in relation to the larger state mental-hygiene system. It depends for its resources on the plans presented by the Mental Hygiene Commissioner and his staff to the state legislature, and then on the political decisions made by the legislature in appropriating and allocating funds for services. A psychiatric center is related to its local community and, in fact, according to Mental Hygiene law (Article 7.7, Mental Hygiene Laws Chapter 251, as amended to 14 April 1978) a commissioner cannot close a facility without the express consent of the state legislature. One can safely say that the legislature reserves that prerogative to itself in part because such facilities are so important to local economies. Changes that effect the economic well-being of a local community involve the political system.

A state psychiatric-facility director is charged by law (Article 7.21) to appoint and remove employees and officers of the facility, to manage the facility, and to administer its personnel system. However, these powers are constrained by civil-service law and regulation and by union agreements that may be in force. The director is also responsible for the humane care of patients. He exercises supervision and directs the care and treatment of all patients in the facility. The commissioner of mental hygiene, however, promulgates standards and regulations for patient care, and the director is ultimately responsible to the commissioner. While a psychiatric-center director has broad discretion, in the sense that details of care and treatment are left largely to his judgment, the center director is constrained to act within the policies and procedures of the larger mental-hygiene system. Any change effort must also take into account the concerns of the larger system.

Current mental-hygiene law asserts the policy that good patient care is best carried out in community-based settings. "It is the policy of the state of New York that all of its residents who are disabled will receive services according to their individual needs and, whenever possible, in their home communities, to enable them to realize their fullest potential for self fulfillment and independent living in society" (*McKinney's Consolidated Laws of New York,* Annotated Book 34A, 1978, p. 3). Current law (Article 41) also states that it is New York State policy to encourage local governments to develop preventive, rehabilitative, and treatment services in order to provide continuity of care. The unified-services provision of the act (Article 41) indicates the legislative intent to create a local and state partnership in the provision of services in the community. In addition to services provided by state and local governments, the mental-hygiene act gives explicit recognition to the role of the private sector in providing services. Private-sector agencies are included in the partnership. The act recognizes that local government may contract with private agencies for state-reimbursable services, and it gives the private agencies the right to appeal to the commissioner of mental hygiene in the event of disagreements with local-government unit-service directors.

This is not the place to discuss the merits and deficiencies of the current mental-hygiene law. It is sufficient to point out that the law itself recognizes the complex community-service environment, and it recognizes the need for cooperation among the diverse service elements. Note that if a state psychiatric-facility director is to proceed with state mandates to promote community-based treatment and rehabilitation programs, then the director must necessarily interact with the local service community. Any change strategy directed toward community-based treatment must necessarily take the local community's service structure into account.

Given the complex context within which any social change takes place, a change agent has much to take into account simultaneously. The change strategy must concern itself with patients, staff, mental-hygiene officials, state legislators, local government officials, service providers in the private sector, and, since patients are to be discharged to local communities and treated there, the attitudes of citizens. The change effort must not only concern itself with the reallocation of human and material resources to new functions but it must also concern itself with people's feelings and attitudes as well. In what follows, we shall describe how Haveliwala's change strategy took all these issues into account.

Clear Goals and Objectives

The director knew what he wanted to do. He had very clear goals and objectives in mind. He intended to reduce the hospital census while making provision for humane care of high quality inside and outside the hospital. He also intended to preserve the center, if not the hospital, by extending its services and embedding them into the complex resource networks existing in communities in the center's catchment area. Recall that Harlem Valley was threatened with closing. Since the center was the primary source of employment for many in that rural area, employees were motivated to continue its life. The director recognized the economic significance of the center to its employees in his statement of goals. Those objectives were repeatedly restated beginning in the first EC meeting. He left no doubt in anyone's mind about what was to be the first priority. Having articulated clear goals, the director used them to maintain motivation at moments of crisis or to rationalize choices. Others could see that choices were reasonable in pursuit of the goals and not capricious or determined by personal favoritism.

The director presented the goals in a framework of moral and professional values. Deinstitutionalization provided better care for patients and was in keeping with good, contemporary practice as well as with New York State policy, as expressed by the legislature. Moreover, interest in the preservation of the psychiatric center served the interests of patient welfare as well. Outpatient services had to be provided by someone if patients were not to be abandoned. Since the center intended to prevent hospitalization as well, it had to develop new services targeted toward unserved high-risk groups. (These goals are also mentioned in New York State mental-hygiene law.) Employees were willing to struggle to achieve highly valued goals. The value framework also provided a morally defensible position against attack by others with conflicting interests.

Establishing Authority through the Willingness to Take Action

The director's first important action took place immediately on assuming office. He proposed and implemented an important change. By taking action rapidly, he made it clear that he was going to act and that he was not going to be bound by what existed. By implementing the new EC immediately, he downgraded the authority and status of several who participated in the older, larger EC. He signaled his willingness to bypass traditional lines of authority within the institution. A department head who ordinarily would have had authority to assign personnel might not have ever been consulted about changing a staff member's unit assigment. The degree of firmness of his intention to support the new structure did not become clear until it was tested in various ways, but his willingness to take action even when the actions were likely to prove unpopular was demonstrated immediately.

Actions as Rational and Related to Goals and Objectives

The reorganization of the EC was rationally related to the overall goals of the organization. The change was designed to facilitate other changes. The purpose of the reorganization was to place more authority into the hands of those responsible for implementing clinical programs. The unit chiefs were responsible for placing patients and developing community-based services. If they were to be held accountable for results, then it made sense that they should participate in making decisions. The unit chiefs had to be able to deploy personnel as their own programs required.

The reorganization placed the unit chiefs between department heads and staff who would ordinarily report through them. The director supported the change. He literally ignored some of his department chiefs. He minimized their responsibilities, even if it meant that some people were left with few duties and were receiving salaries for doing very little. It became clear to all that employees in different departments would have to respect the new interdisciplinary unit and team structure. He used his administrative powers to promote changes that would prepare the organization to meet its new objectives.

The drastic change in social organization was subordinate to clear organizational aims. The reorganization was designed to provide unit-level personnel with more authority and flexibility in carrying out assignments. The unit and team structure motivated many staff who were pleased with the new egalitarianism that characterized their functioning. However, the egalitarian atmosphere was not simply developed for its own sake. Rather it was developed because it seemed the best way to get the job done. Similarly, the units were reorganized several times, and reporting lines were changed. Sometimes one unit chief had responsibility for both inpatient and outpatient services. Later as outpatient services developed, it seemed more appropriate to have outpatient and inpatient unit chiefs, with liaison personnel. Still later the reduced inpatient census required another reorganization to take into account changed responsibilities. Harlem Valley reorganized a number times in the four years. Each reorganization was designed to make the structure functional for accomplishing its goals at that time. Reorganization was not introduced simply to shake things up, but rather it was purposefully designed to solve organizational problems.

Openness, Responsibility, Accountability, and Peer Pressure

Reorganization helped solve the problem of how to deal with personnel who were opposed to change for whatever reason, or temperamentally unsuited to work in the new community-oriented programs. Given civil-service and union regulations, the director knew he had little power to hire and fire at will. He also viewed himself as temperamentally unsuited to move people by a process of counseling and slow persuasion. He decided to use peer pressure and social accountability as the forces to motivate change. The EC not only became a deliberative and decision-making body; it also became a public forum within which each unit chief's success and failure in achieving objectives was reviewed.

The process worked as follows. Each unit chief was asked to consult with staff and to produce and justify target numbers of patients who could be placed in appropriate community settings by a given date. Each unit chief presented these targets, with justifications for them, in the EC meeting. Generally speaking, the director would ask for more than the unit chief offered to produce.

Once objectives were assigned, unit chiefs would be held accountable for meeting them. After it was in place, the program-evaluation division regularly provided quantitative data showing how well each unit met its target. Each unit chief was responsible for presenting and explaining the unit's program-evaluation report (see program evaluation section that follows). All data were available to all EC members and to many others as well. The EC meeting minutes were widely distributed inside and outside the center (for example, to the regional director of the New York State Mental Hygiene Department). If the targets were not being met, the unit chief had to explain why.

Data were widely available. Failure was public. Some unit chiefs were able to meet and even exceed their targets. Their success created competitive pressure. The requirement to explain and discuss evaluation reports made it more difficult for unit chiefs to hide behind invalid excuses. Other unit chiefs recognized excuses. So did the associate director, Von Holden, who had faced the same problems himself as a unit chief. Data from the quality-assurance program, the quality-of-care program (see quality-assurance and quality-of-care sections that follow), and from other monitoring devices are employed in exactly the same way. Unit chiefs are responsible for explaining publically the reasons for deficits in their programs and are accountable for correcting deficiencies.

Creative Use of Competitive Pressure

The system in which each unit is held publically accountable for its own data and for its own performance can generate its own tensions, if for no other reason than that Americans are competitive, and ambitious Americans are highly sensitive to competitive advantage and disadvantage. Even small differences in performance can make large differences in feelings. In this situation several unit chiefs had comparable tasks and were held publically accountable for results. It is easy to see how competitive pressures were generated that drove the whole organization to greater effort.

The system can be likened to one in which there are a number of oscillators (the unit chiefs), controlling production units, each sensitive to the vibration frequency of the fastest one. As one oscillator increases its frequency, reflecting greater activity, the other oscillators are stimulated to greater motion as well. If the other oscillators (the unit chiefs) transmit the message to the units they govern that greater activity is required, then the fastest oscillator, the pacesetter, tends to drive the whole system. Since the director approved intense performance and since he allocated resources and rewards based on performance, the director acted to stimulate faster rates of activity. Such a system could easily get out of control if it were driven to an ever more furious pace, except that the director also acted as a governor. At some points, he seemed to agree that limits had been reached, and the system's furious pace would be moderated.

The mechanical analogy perhaps helps us to understand something of the way in which open information and accountability introduced competitive pressure that increased the motivation to perform. Earlier Von Holden had played the role of the pacesetting oscillator, the unit chief who exceeded all performance standards, and thereby made all others look bad. Later when Von Holden became associate director, another unit chief seemed to pick up the role of pacesetter. Despite changing personnel and changing assignments, the overall system generated the same tension toward performance. Later when the tasks changed and more patients were seen on an outpatient basis, the task became one of following discharged clients on an outpatient basis, or controlling readmissions, or generating enough other clients in the community to rationalize the amount of staff assigned to outpatient services.

Creative tensions are generated in still another way. The director tends to give more than one person responsibility for developing or investigating a new project. Sometimes the assignments are overlapping, and sometimes the people involved may not be fully aware that another person is working on a similar assignment. All are aware that many projects are in various stages of development at the same time. Within limits, to take advantage of opportunities, the director tends to give rewards and to allocate resources on the basis of the rapidity with which a project is ready for implementation, provided that project has sufficiently high priority in his current plan for development. It often happens that a person who investigates and plans a project will receive responsibility for carrying it out, increasing that individual's domain. Since all are aware of each other's successes and failures, because of the system of open accountability, competitive pressure is continuously generated.

To achieve an organizational aim, the director has been willing to modify lines of authority, bypass the existing organizational structure, and reallocate resources. Although the director is clearly in charge and although he supports his leadership in their agreed upon functions, he does not insist that the organizational chart be observed when it comes to program development. Those who were unable to function within such a fluid structure have either left the organization or have contented themselves with accepting lower statuses. No one has been fired or reduced in civil-service pay grade for failure to fulfill a mission, but people have lost favor, and therefore lost influence, with their peers. As the director said, "I didn't have to fire deadwood." He was willing to use peer pressure to achieve change, and he was willing to make functional changes in the organization even if it meant bypassing the formal organization structure.

Managing Tensions

Competitive pressures and open accountability have not led to cutthroat tactics and to enduring enmities. The remaining executives and middle managers maintain cordial and mutually respectful relationships. Many, but not all, who left retained friendships in the organization. How were the tensions managed?

The staff characterize the director as extraordinarily task oriented. His major concern is getting the job done. He is not given to small talk, nor does he generally express any interest in the personal lives of his staff except as it might relate to business. He is not given to praising staff. Although all recognize that some individuals are more in favor than others, no one ever accuses the director of personal favoritism. If someone is in favor, it is because that individual is productive in meeting the organization's (that is, the director's) goals.

Meetings are rarely characterized by an exploration of feelings nor are feelings expressed for their own sake. The director encourages individuals to question each other and himself and may even relish argument; but the expression of personal feelings is not relevant in this context. Some of his staff have come to believe that the director views emotionally based conflicts and anxieties in his staff as weaknesses. He himself says that he has no one on whom to unburden his feelings and he therefore expects his staff to cope with their anxieties as well. While the director may not appear to encourage the expression of feelings, when crises arise, staff report that he is invariably supportive. A staff member facing a problem can count on careful hearing and on a sound response to the objective characteristics of the situation. The director pressures others to achieve goals, but he rarely seems to express anger at task-oriented opposition to his proposals. He also seems very concerned about fitting the person to the task, thus not asking people to work over their heads.

The system does not make direct provision for working out feelings, and informal mechanisms have arisen. Staff have learned to work out their differences among themselves, and not to allow problems coming from bruised egos or ruffled feathers to reach the director. Von Holden as associate director and Faruki as deputy director, clinical, very often provided emotional support for personnel whose feelings had been hurt when their projects or ideas had been rejected, or when they had been bypassed. Now staff support each other.

The director's task orientation has given rise to a "win some, lose some" philosophy among staff. Rejection of a proposition is not taken as a personal rebuff. Staff have learned the director's "no" may change at another time, and some staff have learned to create conditions that will help them move the director to acquiesce in a program they wish to pursue.

A norm of fair competition seems to have developed. People would not act underhandedly, staff say, and they do not see it as a problem. One of the key people reported that early on, when that individual and another seemed headed for a competitive clash, the two confronted each other, and arrived at an open agreement to fight hard, but to fight fair. Others indicate that there is a norm of competent productivity. If a staff member attempted to violate the norm and to present paper accomplishments that were unwarranted, the person would shortly lose standing.

Two-Way Communication

The director was the driving force, but he knew he had to keep himself open to negative feedback in order to avoid serious error. For that reason, he wanted the decision-making process to be open. He also believed that secrecy bred suspicions and unnecessary discontent. Openness forced individuals to acknowledge their responsibilities. He adopted a number of devices to ensure a two-way flow of communication.

Aware that the EC would not take itself seriously as a decision-making body unless he did, he insisted that all important decisions be discussed in the EC before they were made. Whenever EC members would come to him with a proposal, he would insist that it be discussed in the EC. Even though Haveliwala retained final authority, and even though he frequently had his own ideas, he applied the same principles to himself. Although he is difficult to sway, he encourages debate and listens carefully before he arrives at a final decision. Sometimes he will modify his ideas in relation to what he learns. When he rejects arguments or proposals, he always provides specific reasons for his decision.

He circulated the EC minutes widely in order that others might alert him to possible difficulties. He sent EC minutes and other documents to the regional office, not to seek guidance but to keep the regional director informed. In general, the regional director was supportive of the new thrusts. Haveliwala's door was open to anyone who wished to see him. Employees did not have to go through channels to make appointments with him. He read committee reports, carbons of correspondence, and other documents to keep himself fully informed. Staff say it seems as if he read and remembered everything that was ever sent to him.

Sometimes a staff member would have difficulty speaking forthrightly. His close friend, Deputy Director Faruki served, not unwillingly, to convey messages. His executive coordinator, Louise Hubbard, served a vital linking function in maintaining two-way communication. She understood the director's priorities and could help others time and shape their proposals. She could also help the director understand staff problems.

Haveliwala was insistent that ways be found to implement programs. He refused to accept no for an answer. When told it was against the rules, he insisted on being shown the rules involved. Aware of the pressure he was putting on others to bend rules and aware of the danger of actually violating laws or regulations or that his pressure might cause others to violate laws or regulations to please him, he recognized that he too would need checks and balances. His deputy director, administration, Wendy Acrish, and his business officer, Margaret Grant, provided the checks and balances. Both provided the balance Haveliwala sought to ensure that the system for accountability functioned properly. In the enthusiasm for the rapid development of new programs, it is all too easy for adherence to rules, regulations, and laws to be lost.

Even though Haveliwala wanted action quickly, he consciously limited the pressure he applied to his business officer and to his deputy director, administration, in order to preserve the system of organizational checks and balances. (They may not agree that he pressured with restraint.) As he did with other employees who raised realistic problems in relation to any plan, sometimes he acquiesced to their views. At other times he would continue to insist. On occasion he would accept direct responsibility by signing or countersigning orders. By being open to objection to specific plans, he allowed his colleagues to protect him from grievous error.

Reaching Line Employees

The cooperation of line employees is vital to the success of a change effort in an institution. Unit chiefs had responsibility for implementing decisions and could use any legitimate means at their disposal.

Many of the successful unit chiefs extended the approach within their own teams. Decisions made at the EC were communicated through the EC minutes, and in unit and team meetings held as quickly as possible after the decision had been reached. The unit chiefs and team leaders sought guidance from line personnel about prospective programs. Feedback was sought only within the parameters of the goals that had been established. These were not negotiable. Goals were presented with clarity and firmness to line personnel. Effective unit chiefs conveyed policies in vivid, concrete images understandable to line personnel who may be put off by jargon. Methods were subject to discussion at this level, but not goals.

The team approach required that members give each other feedback. It required that an aide be free to tell a physician that one of his orders had adverse consequences. It also required that supervisors be able to give aids feedback concerning their performance without eliciting defensiveness. Formal feedback devices (program-evaluation reports, quality-assurance and quality-of-care reports) required that units discuss their performance in order to correct deficiencies.

These tasks required that unit chiefs and team leaders be able to develop atmospheres supportive of two-way communication across status lines. Unit chiefs followed the same method of assigning tasks to team leaders, holding the team leaders accountable to them for results, but leaving the methods open. Since the unit accepted responsibility for its total program, the organizational structure discouraged negative use of the concept "it's not my job." Effective unit chiefs and team leaders developed a team spirit.

To help create team spirit, individuals are made to feel important. People are fitted to jobs or jobs suitable to a given individual's skills and temperament are created. Unit chiefs compete to attract talented people in order to get a job done. Unit chiefs occasionally negotiate with each other about the assignment of personnel, much as big league managers might trade athletes to fill a specific need on their teams. (Some employees resented what seemed to them to be behind-closed-doors wheeling and dealing. In subsequent years the "slave trade" was less blatant, and employees were consulted to a greater extent.) Employees selected in this fashion are motivated to work at their strengths. Moreover, since assignments to work out of title can be made only with the employee's consent, those who took on special assignments were interested in the jobs. They were selected because of their talents, and unit chiefs and team leaders encouraged initiative and creativity to make full use of employee talents.

Not all people are interested in challenge, and not all function well with freedom. Many individuals work better with definite assignments, carried out on a regular schedule. Many line employees do not have career ambitions. For some, a steady, secure job was sufficient. Others held second jobs and needed a steady routine.

To take into account the needs of those who were not motivated by challenges or freedom, Harlem Valley developed a series of policy and program manuals. Accepting the idea that many line employees were oriented to obey people in authority, Harlem Valley used that feature of employee culture to mandate changes. Each unit has its own policy and procedures manual, developed in consultation with the employees. The policy and procedures manuals spell out the purposes of each treatment unit and precisely define specific tasks. Where therapy tasks call for new skills, Harlem Valley uses its inservice education program to prepare employees to take on their responsibilities. The unit manuals are supplemented by general policy manuals, written in simple English and readily available on the wards. These manuals spell out the operations of each service in unambiguous terms. They serve as guidelines for employees and are related to the accountability systems in use in the institution.

There are a number of mechanisms for monitoring services and introducing accountability within this system. The quality-assurance program is one of these. It uses standards that were developed in consultation with the units and that are directly related to the specific functions of each unit.

Communication between the Director and Line Staff

The director does not meet regularly with line staff. In fact, it is one of their complaints that the director is a distant figure. Haveliwala did hold a few large "town meetings," but he felt that they were ineffective, and he discontinued them. He does not participate in the clinical or in the teaching program to any extent, and he does not often make visits to the inpatient services. He does write a regular column in the center's newspaper. In the past he videotaped an address that was made available on all units and on all shifts.

EC meetings are held at outpatient centers as well as at Wingdale. Local advisory board members are invited to attend EC meetings held at their clinics. He talks with employees at the outpatient services when he visits there. He is careful to meet all new employees during their orientation, and he takes that opportunity to present Harlem Valley's goals and objectives. He makes time for any employee who wishes to see him. The employee does not have to clear an appointment through unit-level supervisory personnel. Employees are guaranteed confidentiality if they bring complaints to his attention.

Line Employees not Reached

Despite efforts to communicate with line employees, to enrich their jobs, and to work toward greater participation, morale is probably poorest among the therapeutic aids and staff nurses on the inpatient services. Rapid changes have required that these employees adapt to change. Team leaders and unit chiefs change frequently. Each leader has a different personal style and makes different demands of employees. Just as a routine is developed and one adapts to the boss's expectations, a change takes place. Employees do not always willingly move to new wards. A change means the employee has to learn to relate to new patients and to learn new therapeutic plans. Some claim the rapid changes have an adverse influence on patient care. Younger, more acutely ill patients are excited by the changes and may act out more or be more able to manipulate staff. The more chronic patients are probably less affected by such personnel changes. Employees feel they do not commit themselves to their jobs as much. They are more reluctant to bring personal possessions to decorate wards. They are less identified with the wards. Either they or the leader may be gone tomorrow.

Most important, inpatient-ward-level staff feel that changes have been made at their expense. Although no one has been fired, paraprofessional positions have less often been replaced, and paraprofessional items have been converted to professional items. Newly hired professionals who have credentials to obtain higher grade levels and higher pay are often inexperienced compared to the paraprofessionals. Paraprofessionals feel that it is they who are teaching the professionals while the professionals get the pay.

Ward-level personnel feel they have been left with the most difficult patients to treat and that their lot has not improved. Although the hospital shows better personnel-to-patient ratios on the inpatient services, ward-level personnel argue that the ratios do not reflect the amount of personnel time going into research, evaluation, training, committee work, and increasing paperwork. It is difficult to get numbers that clearly show the amount of time going into direct and indirect services, and so this complaint is difficult to assess. The complaint exists. Its validity needs examination.

Their complaints may reflect a perception that inpatient services are regarded as less important than outpatient services within the Harlem Valley hierarchy. Inpatient staff feel their work is not fully appreciated by upper-level management. They feel management does not trust them to care for patients responsibly.

Whatever the reasons, and they are undoubtedly complex, ward-level personnel feel they have benefited least by the changes. Of all groups, they are probably most resentful of many of the changes. The fringe benefits of developing Harlem Valley into a model center do not affect them directly. Many cannot move. They cannot take advantage of the institution's reputation to advance their careers. They do not travel at hospital expense to participate in national conferences as professional staff sometimes do. Many are still concerned that the hospital's survival has not been ensured, and that the continued run down in census will eventually lead to the loss of their positions. Although none have been fired and some have been able to transfer into outpatient services, ward-level personnel do not see the continued thrust toward placement of patients into the community and the reallocation of resources to other than direct patient care as serving their interests.

One must distinguish between job satisfaction and job performance. Good leadership, individual conscientiousness, and the various monitoring devices have led to a very good level of patient care. Patient abuse occurs relatively infrequently, and, when it occurs, it is of a less serious variety than in many other institutions. Although a recent JCAH site-visit team recommended more inpatient programming, the program was acceptable and the general level of care considered very good. So far, morale problems have not resulted in poor patient care.

7

A Competency-Based Organization

Formal organizations, particularly those in the public sector, establish educational and experience requirements for entry into given positions. These requirements are intended to introduce quality control in the sense that the best qualified people, as defined by their credentials, are those who are accepted for given positions. The requirements that candidates possess certain credentials and that their credentials be reviewed through a civil-service structure also serves a public purpose. Jobs are presumably filled on the basis of ability and not on the basis of political or personal favoritism. An objective system is necessary in order to maintain a fair system, trusted by the public. To the degree that one's formal credentials do ensure capable performance is the degree to which the public interest is served by the requirement.

In recent years we have seen considerable questioning of the value or the necessity for formal credentials to fill particular positions. The questioning probably began with the antipoverty program that committed itself to hiring indigenous nonprofessional and paraprofessional personnel in a variety of service jobs (Alley and Blanton 1978). However, others have commented that academic training does not necessarily fit one to carry out clinical functions, and clinical training and experience does not necessarily fit one to carry out administrative, managerial, and leadership tasks. We have seen many examples of people from a variety of professions and with no special training do very well in positions for which they had few formal credentials (see Goldenberg 1971). The folk saying has it, "From each group will emerge a leader," and there is some truth in the saying. In undermanned settings, settings in which there are insufficient numbers of people to do the work of the setting, participants do not worry about who will do the job but rather how will the job get done. And the job gets done.

The existence of formal qualifications for entry into given positions, whatever other value it has, restricts the availability of people to do the job to the pool of only those who have the appropriate credentials. However, if one establishes as a credential for entry into a position only the competence to do the job (or the willingness and the ability to learn rapidly), then the pool of potentially talented people increases accordingly. Moreover, if one assumes general managerial and leadership competence and is not constrained by a requirement that people in positions of leadership have specific technical qualifications, then the pool of potential leaders or managers also increases since talented people can be used in a variety of capacities.

Harlem Valley appears to have adopted both assumptions, that of competence rather than status as a requirement for holding a position, and general managerial competence rather than specific technical background, as the key qualification for work assignments. One might say that a key strategy was changing the system from one based on formal credentials and formal status to one based on competence. Within very broad limits, staff hold leadership positions because of their ability to do the job and less because of professional credentials or civil-service grade. Von Holden says the system is based on the principle of making the organizational chart congruent with the organization's informal structure.

The director, who is very task oriented, has used his authority to administer the institution to delegate responsibility and to determine the lines of authority within the institution. The frequently changing organizational chart reflects a flexible, problem-solving approach. Each organizational change was an attempt to solve a problem that the dynamic, changing situation had brought to the fore. The specific changes at any time reflect both the problem to be solved and appraisals of the strengths of personnel available to do the necessary jobs. The organizational chart may also reflect past successes in accomplishing missions since functions may tend to accrue to executives who carried out particular missions. Tailoring jobs to fit people may be considered instances of technostructuring approaches to organizational change.

The ability to move people into different positions is constrained by civil-service requirements. While the director may delegate responsibilities, he cannot give the incumbent the pay and rank that go with the job if the person does not have the appropriate educational and experience credentials to qualify for the civil-service rank. Harlem Valley has found a variety of nonmonetary incentives to reward employees who take on responsibilities beyond those called for in the formal job title and job description that each actually holds. There have been some problems in this approach. These problems include maintaining employee motivation and dealing with the feelings of those who function in supervisory structures in which a subordinate may hold a higher formal civil-service grade than the designated leader of the unit. These will also be described here.

Using the Organizational Chart to Support
Managerial Competence

Some executives seem to worship an organizational chart, as if the chart itself is the key to the solution of organizational problems. A neat organizational chart appears to be an end in and of itself. The organizational chart should reflect the executive's understanding of the nature of the organization and the functions that have to be fulfilled. An organizational chart may be built around the talents of available personnel. In that case it may not be as neat or as symmetrical as one built around some other theory of management, but it may be more likely to reflect the current tasks that have to be accomplished, and it may reflect the executive's understanding that doing a job requires more flexible control over certain resources. In this section we shall provide some examples of the use of organizational titles, lines of reporting, and reorganizations to reflect the talents of individuals.

In the first few months after Haveliwala assumed the directorship, he appointed psychologist Martin Von Holden as *acting* deputy director, clinical, even though Von Holden had neither a medical degree nor a Ph.D. at the time. When Dr. Ghulam Faruki, was appointed deputy director, clinical, Von Holden was appointed associate director, and placed at the same level on the organizational chart as Faruki. The title associate director does not exist in the civil-service system. It was created at Harlem Valley to accommodate a person in order to fulfill a task.

Duties were divided according to each individual's strengths. Faruki had the job of improving medical psychiatric care, improving hospital records, and instituting review mechanisms to guarantee the quality of care. The medical-surgical service and the geriatric service that had a large medical component reported to Faruki. Since most of the unit chiefs were nonmedical people and issues of medical responsibility arose, deputy unit chiefs were invariably physicians. The deputy unit chiefs technically reported through the unit chiefs, but in so far as their medical duties were concerned, they were responsible to Faruki.

Von Holden's job as associate director was to continue to place patients in the community. Unit chiefs reported through Von Holden. Unit chiefs were responsible for identifying patients to be placed, for developing discharge plans, and for developing community-based outpatient services. Many decisions affecting inpatient care went through Von Holden and required careful coordination with Faruki. Von Holden and Faruki, who developed great respect and affection for each other, worked cooperatively to solve problems that arose as a result of the criss-crossing lines of responsibility. Because both responded to clear priorities and kept the good of the total center in mind, they were able to work out effective compromises to get the job done without worrying about considerations of status or professional turf.

Another reorganization took place recently. Earlier both inpatient and outpatient services were under the direction of the same unit chief. As the hospital's inpatient census declined and outpatient services developed, some unit chiefs were given outpatient responsibilities only, and liaisons were designated to help coordinate efforts. With a further decline in the census and with the more elaborate development of outpatient services, problems of coordination developed.

Given the greatly reduced inpatient census, it seemed logical to develop two units with both inpatient and outpatient responsibilities. A chief appropriate for one of the newly proposed units was available. It was more difficult to find a chief for the second unit. The logical candidate pleaded that he had neither the temperament, the skills, nor the desire to fill the position. Because that individual had been doing a good job in his present demanding outpatient assignment, the director, after considering several alternatives within the EC, decided to keep that individual in his present assignment. He appointed an inpatient unit chief with no outpatient responsibilities. The organizational chart is unbalanced, but the positions fit individual competencies and desires.

Currently David Sorenson is associate director. Sorenson is a rehabilitation specialist whose major experience was in the field of mental retardation. Many of the program-development responsibilities that were Von Holden's now are Sorenson's. Sorenson holds the position because the director believes vocational rehabilitation is the therapy of choice for schizophrenic patients who tend to become chronic patients. Sorenson's professional background is appropriate for the center's current direction of development. Sorenson is the executive responsible for many other aspects of the community-support system (for example, living arrangements, day care, workshops, and transportation) partly because he has shown himself to be effective in getting things done and partly because it is necessary to coordinate other aspects of the community-support system with work-oriented programs.

The responsibility for program evaluation is located in one department. Monitoring and evaluating the quality of care, with the additional responsibility of conducting special medical-care evaluation studies and clinically oriented research is located in another department. Epidemiological research is conducted in still another separate department. In some organizations several of these functions might be unified under a single department head. At Harlem Valley the people who are responsible had either developed the programs or had taken them over and improved them. Organizational logic gave way to individual competency in developing the reporting relationships. People with particular aptitudes and talents fill the jobs. Mary Ann Valinski, in charge of the quality-assurance program, is a registered nurse with a title that does not exist in the civil-service lexicon. She is called a "quality-assurance engineer." She holds the position because she does it well.

Steve Witte, assistant to the deputy director, administration, is a clinical social worker. He supervises leased space for outpatient services. He had no formal training for this job. Witte was hired because a clinical line was available and a job needed to be done. Witte had no administrative or business background, but he was willing to learn. His appointment provided an organizational bonus in that a clinical perspective could be represented in the deputy director, administration, office. Deputy director Acrish trained and supervised Witte in his administrative functions, and he is available to advise her on clinical issues that affect administrative decisions.

A Managerial Model

Managerial competence is a requirement for occupying a position of leadership and authority at Harlem Valley. Haveliwala defines managerial competence as the ability to take on a task assignment, to develop a plan for carrying out that assignment, to select, motivate, and supervise employees to carry out the necessary tasks, and to be accountable for producing results.

The managerial model assumes that executive skills transcend the particular assignment. Just as an automobile executive may take a job in food processing, so may a social worker take charge of leasing outpatient space or a registered nurse be charged with overseeing the quality-assurance program.

Harlem Valley has a core group of managers who move among assignments in inpatient and outpatient work, between direct and indirect services. Sometimes people are assigned to jobs, and sometimes they make their own jobs by suggesting projects to the director and the EC. Harlem Valley's atmosphere encourages a fit between person and job, just as the therapeutic program emphasizes a fit between the patient's characteristics and the social environment in which the patient lives and works.

New assignments stimulate renewed interest. A Hawthorne effect is created over and over. Managers do not become jaded on the job. New challenges offer new opportunities to exercise creativity, to develop new competencies, and to leave some old problems behind.

Some individuals find the challenge of new assignments and the demand for performance emotionally exhausting. Some burn out, long for routine, and for the time and energy to pay attention to family and other personal needs. New managers are tested. Some staff members try to use the new manager's inexperience in that setting to subvert hard-won gains. A new manager inherits problems and may need to be the "bad guy" to shape up the operation.

On balance, the managerial concept seems to operate effectively. Harlem Valley has a number of people who can be counted on to undertake new assignments and perform effectively. This group that includes nurses, psychologists, and social workers makes it possible to contemplate new programs with the knowledge that capable individuals are at hand and usually willing. So far, the system has survived despite the departure of key people. New people replace them and seem to adapt.

Physicians and Managers

The problems that emerge when individuals of lesser formal status supervise people of greater status are most acute in the relationship between nonmedical managers and physicians. At the outset it might be stated that the system works because the director is unwavering in support of managerial personnel.

Physicians who were most intolerant of the arrangement left early. The director was not deterred by threats of physicians' leaving. He had confidence in his ability to recruit replacements as necessary. Those hired subsequently were informed of the supervisory arrangements. People who accepted the positions agreed to work within that structure. Day-by-day problems have been worked out, but the issue is always underneath the surface.

Nonmedical managers (registered nurses, social workers, psychologists) supervise physicians. (So far, only clinically trained personnel have filled managerial roles in predominantly clinical units. It remains to be seen whether non-clinically trained personnel can be equally effective.) The arrangement poses problems for both the nonmedical manager and the physician. Formal and informal solutions have emerged.

Unit chiefs have decisional authority while physicians under them have medical responsibility for patient care. Nonmedical unit chiefs have physicians assigned as their deputy unit chiefs. Deputy unit chiefs provide the medical supervision for physicians responsible to nonmedical team leaders. Any disputes are referred to the deputy unit chief. If the unit chief and the deputy unit chief cannot agree, the dispute may be referred to the deputy director, clinical, the highest clinical position in the table of organization. Disputes arose when patients were being released rapidly to the community. At that time unit chiefs frequently differed with physicians about a patient's readiness for release. At present most decisions are reached by concensus. Conflicts rarely arise.

Nonmedical managers are also responsible for supervising physicians' work assignments, their days off, and their completion of paperwork. The difference in status has created some tensions for both supervisors and subordinates. A nurse who supervises the work of a physician must overcome years of conditioning to adopt an authoritative stance vis à vis the physician. Women who fill authority roles find their lives are complicated by sex-role issues, further complicated by the fact that many male physicians are foreign born and unused to working with women who have authority.

A number of compromises support the physician's professional autonomy. Medical personnel still have special status. The By-laws of the Medical Staff accept the concept of nonmedical managers and unit chiefs, but membership on the medical staff is restricted to physicians and dentists. The by-laws explicitly recognize the concept of medical responsibility. Performance evaluations of physicians are conducted by deputy unit chiefs, physicians, and are appealed to the deputy director, clinical, also a physician in the event of differences of opinion. Performance ratings of the deputy unit chiefs are made by the deputy director, clinical.

Dr. Faruki, very skillful in mediating conflicts between the medical and nonmedical staff, met regularly with the physicians. He used the meeting as an opportunity to foster the change process. He did not allow the meeting to become a griping session. It became a teaching session with a focus on modern psychiatric approaches (for example, drugs, contemporary use of electric shock, and therapeutic community). He also used the sessions to explain medical-records audits. The audits became teaching devices to help physicians improve their practices. Dr. Haveliwala also meets with the medical staff, reinforcing their identification with him.

Staff are unanimous in agreeing that at the level of the assignment of responsibility or the allocation of resources, the director has shown no favoritism to medical over nonmedical personnel. He has maintained his task-oriented approach in that delicate area. Decisions are based on performance, on his view of priorities, or the opportunities to achieve a particular goal, but not on personal favoritism or formal status.

Nonmonetary Incentives and the Selection of Personnel

Harlem Valley makes extensive use of nonmonetary incentives to provide for employees who take on responsibility beyond that called for by their job descriptions. By "nonmonetary incentive," we mean anything of psychological or material value other than direct cash payment. Nonmonetary incentives do use budget since employees are being paid to fulfill certain functions, but no additional cash is required.

Budgetary constraints and civil-service requirements place limits on the ability of a center director to offer direct monetary incentives. There are no cash bonuses for performance. Employees can be promoted, but they must meet educational and experience requirements for the higher grade, independently of their competence to perform the work. A center is allocated only so many lines or items at different grade levels. The desired grade level may not be available at the time the employee is ready for promotion.

In order to generate a high degree of commitment, Harlem Valley had to select people for whom the conditions of work were rewarding and for whom other incentives were meaningful. Harlem Valley employed the principle of good people selecting good people successfully. One cannot help but be impressed with the energy, the intelligence, the diligence, and the competence with which many of the upper- and middle-level managers go about their jobs. Program plans and other documents are well thought through, highly detailed, and well written. Perusing various archives, one is impressed with the sheer volume of high-quality work completed in a relatively short period of time. It is obvious that many are very good at what they do.

Competence, however, is not the only principle of selection. Many of the key executives had had two or more years of experience in similar programs before they came to Harlem Valley. One might say they had made their mistakes elsewhere and had learned from them. What at first glance seems superior wisdom may well be the scars of battle. The key people were not just out of school. They had worked in the types of programs they were now to implement on a larger scale. Such people were attracted by the possibility of putting into practice ideas that were not as fully implemented elsewhere.

Harlem Valley also made it a point to select people who were interested in professional advancement. Almost all the key people were individuals who were ambitious professionally or who had long-term interests in careers in the state system. Professionally ambitious people understand that participation in well-regarded innovative programs will advance their careers.

The people who accepted the acting roles and non-civil-service titles, although receiving pay commensurate with their permanent civil-service grades, found it to their advantage to work out of title. Some did it to grow personally or for the excitement inherent in the enterprise. Some enjoyed the prestige, status, and power that went with the role. Some were intrigued by the idea that in filling particular roles (for example, unit chiefs) and supervising people of higher status (for example, physicians), they were doing something that was unusual and groundbreaking in their own profession. Beyond the psychological advantage, documented supervisory experience helped the individual to qualify for a higher civil-service grade.

Some were promised they would get the higher level civil-service grade as soon as it was available and they were eligible for it. For some, such promotions came relatively quickly. For others, promotions were delayed. Sometimes the item would not be approved by civil service. Sometimes the individual's experience or educational qualifications were deemed insufficient. Sometimes an available higher grade item was used to recruit a person from outside. Some individuals resented what was perceived, rightly or wrongly, as a broken promise. Some individuals felt promotions were dangled before them as carrots to manipulate them. Those who received the promotions within a reasonable time were exceedingly pleased. Those who felt they had labored long and hard without receiving just rewards felt hurt. On balance, for most, the rewards of the position were sufficient to compensate for the lack of money to go along with the position.

Other rewards were available. Some obtained excellent, subsidized housing on the hospital's grounds. For some, the feeling of being in the inner circle, closest to the director, was a reward. Some were rewarded with educational leaves. Others obtained trips to conventions. The hospital did not require that executives account for hours or punch a time clock. Executives followed the professional pattern of working as many hours as necessary to do a job, and then taking time off, as circumstances permitted on an hour-by-hour basis. Many valued that freedom.

Harlem Valley tried to provide tangible rewards for its employees. Its catchment area extends over 70 miles. Each day teams traveled from the hospital to staff community-based programs. In order to get in a full day in the community-based center, some workers elected a ten-hour day, four days a week. Travel time was counted as work time. The compensation of flexible working hours made it worthwhile for many. Later the practice was stopped when the state as employer insisted that travel to and from a work site could not be considered work time. The issue was compromised by allowing half the time as work time, but some of the motivation was lost.

8

Evaluation, Feedback, and the Spirit of Inquiry

Harlem Valley makes extensive use of evaluative and monitoring devices to assess the degree to which programs are achieving objectives, the degree to which standards of quality are being maintained, and to contribute to management decisions. Information is collected systematically. It is widely distributed, and it is used. The director, unit chiefs, and heads of departments all receive information and are accountable for correcting deficits in programs revealed by the various evaluative devices. When program decisions are made, resources are allocated in relation to measured workload and in relation to program objectives set in accord with institution priorities. When evaluative and monitoring devices reveal programmatic problems, special studies are undertaken. Most important, the director has shown his executives that he does rely heavily on data so they also use evaluation information in planning and reviewing their own efforts. The use of evaluation and monitoring devices may be considered examples of data-based change strategies. The development of a spirit of inquiry is consistent with the organizational development objective of creating an organizational culture conducive to flexible problem solving.

The Spirit of Inquiry

The director fosters a spirit of inquiry. The spirit of inquiry refers to the scientific attitude in which hypotheses are held subject to test by data. The best example may be found in the way in which Dr. Haveliwala speaks of the objective of deinstitutionalizing and developing community-based services. Although in his public posture as a leader, he is absolutely firm and unbending in his support of the deinstitutionalization objective, his private convictions are more open. He is fully aware of contemporary thinking about mental illness and the limits of our knowledge. However, he argues that given the state of the mental-health art, judging from his own clinical experience, and judging from the research literature, community-based methods are no less adequate than other methods. Community-based treatment may well have additional beneficial effects on both patients and communities. His position is a rational one, tied to existing empirical evidence, and presumably open to modification with additional evidence.

The spirit of inquiry is manifested in his argument that even imperfect data are better than no data in informing decisions. The desire for data implies that all programmatic efforts are tentative, subject to modification as data indicates a need for change. He intends for his decisions to be data based as much as possible. Although other considerations also enter into programmatic decisions, the variety of evaluative and research services bring data, however imperfect, into the forefront of discussion about programs.

Program Evaluation

Psychologist Paula Wolfe, who had worked with Haveliwala at South Beach, was one of the first new employees he recruited. She was assigned to develop an automated program-evaluation system that would allow each unit to track each patient on a regular basis. At Harlem Valley, the term "program evaluation" refers to statistical information concerning the demographic characteristics of the patients served, and indicators of the service rendered such as the number of admissions, the services each client received, the length of stay, the number of discharged clients followed in outpatient settings, and the rate of broken appointments in outpatient settings. [The extensive program evaluation literature cannot be cited here. A good discussion of the use of program evaluation in management contexts in mental health centers can be found in Hagedorn, Beck, Neupert, and Werlin, (1976).] Special follow-up studies of the current status of discharged cohorts are undertaken from time to time. Data are collected by the unit that provides the service, and they are evaluated in relation to objectives that were established for each program in discussion in the EC. Reports are provided on varying time schedules, some monthly and some quarterly. Special studies and special reports are also compiled and presented as the need arises.

Wolfe, who had been a program evaluator at South Beach, worked with several principles (Wolfe and Haveliwala 1976). Her approach was practical. She consulted with unit chiefs to work out goals and measurable behavioral objectives for program evaluation. She was not interested in elaborate experimental designs or elegant indices but rather in getting useful, timely information, appropriate for decision making. If program-evaluation data were to be useful in management decisions, she had to be ready to modify the program-evaluation system as the organization changed. Software was developed anticipating changes. To minimize disruption, she intended as much as possible to use data already being collected. She also wanted a decentralized staff. Therefore, each unit appointed a medical-records clerk responsible for collecting program-evaluation data. The clerks also collected data required for state reports or for utilization review. Clerks were trained to use a detailed checklist for data collection and tabulation so that errors could be kept to a minimum.

She requested that unit chiefs present their own data at the EC meetings. That way each had to know the data, and in effect "owned" them. That simple tactic provided leverage in reducing resistance to filling out forms. If a record clerk noticed that forms were missing, the record clerk on the service would speak to that individual directly or to the unit chief. Because the unit chiefs had a stake in the data, they would act to correct problems. At present there is very little resistance to providing data. The current program evaluation director, Dr. Marge Braeren, states that relatively few data are lost or misreported.

Wolfe believes, as do others, that program evaluation is important at Harlem Valley because Dr. Haveliwala takes it seriously. He studies the data, uses them in his discussions with others, and insists that others use data for planning or to justify changes. As program evaluator, she participated in the EC meetings and worked to use data not to clobber people but as a point of departure for discussion and correction of problems.

As program evaluator, Wolfe also participated on various center committees, including one responsible for placement review. As a member of the placement-review committee, she made site visits. She obtained firsthand knowledge of the settings in which patients were placed. That direct experience brought her out of the "ivory tower" and helped her to understand the significance of the numbers in evaluation reports.

As with all other programs at Harlem Valley, program evaluation is also subject to review and modification. Unit chiefs and other executives comment on the usefulness of the procedures, on problems that develop, and on the need for new information as situations change. These reviews lead to change in program-evaluation procedures in order to keep it relevant.

As program evaluator, Wolfe was close to the director and participated in key executive meetings. After she left to take a position in the regional office, the person who followed her evidently attempted to change some of the procedures and in the process produced conflict. During that period program-evaluation data were less useful, and the program evaluator had less influence in the decision-making process. Dr. Braeren has been able to maintain the system and is now working to develop outcome and follow-up studies in addition to studies that monitor ongoing programs. Program-evaluation reports continue to be taken seriously, especially when budgetary issues require careful attention to program development.

Quality Assurance

The quality-assurance program has been in existence for about two and one half years. Its purpose is to guarantee that standards of service are being met. There are currently 37 programs that are reviewed on a weekly basis. These include all patient units and support services such as the patient canteen, housekeeping, and the business office. Each program developed a checklist of observables that enables an evaluator to determine, within a half-hour's visit, whether or not the service was properly doing its job. Standards were developed by each service, but they cannot be set too low because they are reviewed by the director and EC before being accepted. The checklist of observables for a ward, for example, include items such as:

1. The telephone is answered within five rings. The person speaking and the service is properly identified.
2. The ward physician can be located within 10 minutes.
3. No patients are lying on the floor.
4. Attendants are speaking to patients.
5. Therapy aids can describe the major purpose of the service.

The checklist of observables for the canteen include such items as:

1. Customers are served promptly (within 3 minutes).
2. Customers are addressed politely.
3. Counter attendants are neatly dressed.
4. Packaged foods have current freshness dates.
5. Storerooms are locked.

Each service is visited once a week by an executive from some other division. The service does not know who is assigned to visit, nor when the person will visit. No service is evaluated by its own personnel. Each evaluator submits a report to Mary Ann Valinski, the quality-assurance engineer. Quantitative scores reflecting compliance with standards are distributed weekly to the services involved, to the unit chiefs, to other members of the EC, and to the director. Monthly summaries showing trends are also distributed. If a service falls below standard, its head is responsible for correcting the deficit. Subsequent reports show whether or not the deficit has been corrected.

Dr. Haveliwala instituted an award of the month for the program that has shown the greatest improvement in the previous three months. The winning unit receives a certificate. Dr. Haveliwala will meet with the unit in an informal get together, enabling individuals to interact with him on their grounds rather than in his office.

The evaluation process is under continual review. Evaluators are sometimes lax in applying the criteria. However, the aim is to maintain scores in the 80-90-percent range. If a unit begins to attain scores of 100 percent regularly, criteria are revised.

Quality assurance serves at least two purposes. First, it puts eyes on all the services and provides a form of mutual criticism. If one can argue that bad things go on in institutions because of a conspiracy of silence, then the quality-assurance program establishes a norm of criticizing unacceptable practices and correcting them. Line personnel sometimes say they do not need the quality-assurance program to motivate them to provide good care, but they also say it keeps them on their toes.

Second, because the quality-assurance program draws its evaluators from managers in all disciplines and services, all managers obtain firsthand contact with parts of the center they would not ordinarily see. It enables people to have a somewhat more sympathetic appreciation of each other's jobs and problems. It is one thing for a personnel officer to read a job description. It is another thing to observe a ward attendant clean an incontinent patient.

The quality-assurance program is used in the same way as other data systems, to provide information to all about the state of all services. The open distribution of information produces competitive motivation to maintain standards of service throughout the institution. It is difficult to determine the precise effect of quality assurance since no baseline data were collected before the system was installed. It may be that it is superficial and may miss some critical failures in service delivery. Instances of patient abuse do come up from time to time. Evidently the quality-assurance mechanism does not eliminate such problems entirely. On its face, it is a distinct effort to maintain standards of care systematically, and it is part of the elaborate system of feedback used to keep the institution on course.

Quality-Care Program

The quality-care program began with the necessity to update medical records and to institute peer-review systems to meet accreditation, insurance, and Medicare-Medicaid-reimbursement requirements. It began under the direction of Dr. Ghulam Faruki and has been used as a means of upgrading the level of care in the hospital and upgrading the quality of medical records. The office has been directed by Dr. Chung Moon since 1976.

The quality-care program contributes to several aspects of the total program. First, it acts as a control over the quality of care. It does this through reviewing ongoing medical records against standards established for the quality of treatment and the adequacy of the record. When deficiencies are uncovered in medical records, individual therapists as well as unit chiefs are given explicit feedback. The individual therapist is required to make a written response to the critique. When corrective action is indicated, responsiveness is monitored.

Second, it performs a teaching function. The central review committee has representatives from each of the service units. In reviewing and evaluating records, the representatives learn the standards of care. In theory, they feed back their learning to others on their service not only to improve record keeping but also to improve the care implied in the record keeping.

Third, the office of quality care establishes criteria for admission, discharge, and placement. The utilization-review process is used to ascertain that new admissions have been properly screened; that appropriate criteria for hospitalization have been followed when a patient is hospitalized; that treatment plans are formulated rapidly; and that treatment plans are followed, or if inadequate, modified. Utilization-review data contribute to the program-evaluation system and enter into management decisions. Beyond ensuring appropriate patient care, utilization review uncovers clinical problems. If the numbers of admissions are high, the particular unit chief is required to explain. The explanation might lead to a decision to develop an additional mobile crisis team or a hospital-diversion unit in the community to avoid formal hospitalization. This year the office has established utilization-review criteria for patients in the various levels of outpatient programs and in domiciliary-care settings. An outpatient utilization-review coordinator has been assigned to each outpatient service to carry out ongoing review. These reviews are used to see that patients do not remain in a placement but are moved along to more independent-living circumstances as soon as they seem able to progress.

Fourth, the quality-care program feeds into the research program in the spirit of inquiry. The central utilization review committee initiates medical-care-evaluation studies. These studies indicate the need for new programs or for inservice education to correct problem areas. An example will suffice. Review of records indicated that two or more psychotropic drugs were used concomitantly in a large proportion of cases. The study was followed by an inservice education program to alert the medical staff to problems in the use of combinations of drugs. Subsequent studies showed that prescriptions of multiple drugs declined.

A number of other studies deriving from utilization-review procedures have been completed. These include a review of the characteristics of patients with multiple admissions, review of length of stay, and a review of characteristics of patients admitted from correctional institutions. These special clinical studies are widely distributed, presented in the EC meetings, and considered for their implications for the development of programs. When changes are indicated, unit chiefs have the responsibility to institute appropriate corrective action.

The office of quality of care has responsibility for setting and adopting standards and monitoring clinical practices. These responsibilities are fulfilled through a centralized utilization-review committee, through the system of decentralized utilization-review coordinators and through medical-care-evaluation studies that are undertaken by the office when particular questions emerge. Each utilization-review coordinator is responsible to the unit chief. The inpatient medical-records and utilization-review committees and appropriate subcommittees meet on a biweekly basis. The comparable outpatient groups meet on a monthly basis. There is also a utilization-review coordinators' meeting biweekly. Problems in the system are reviewed in these meetings.

The separation of the office of quality care from the office of program evaluation presents some problems of coordination and cooperation. The problem of integrating individual-care review data with overall program reviews is yet to be solved. As we have indicated, a great deal of data is collected, although all who collect data attempt to use the existing record system as much as possible. Designated record clerks and utilization-review coordinators complete the various forms, but sometimes they need to go to clinical personnel for additional information. From time to time the research office undertakes studies that require information from personnel. The office of quality care has recently introduced a problem-oriented medical record. These complicated forms require additional training and require additional time to complete. The several offices have to cooperate in order to get information appropriate to each one's needs and without overloading the system with requests for data. These are operational problems that stem from the way in which offices develop at Harlem Valley. All are aware of the problems, and as far as we can tell, the several professionals make the effort to cooperate.

Epidemiology

About three years ago, Dr. Roger Christenfeld joined Harlem Valley as a consultant in epidemiology, working two to three days a week. He is responsible for developing epidemiological data for Harlem Valley's geographic districts. He has undertaken special studies on clinically relevant topics (for example, the geographic clustering of patients), follow-up studies of patients placed in the community, and needs-assessment studies of special populations (for example, adolescents in one county). Unit chiefs use his data to assess future program needs and to negotiate with local human-service agencies to develop appropriate services.

Dr. Christenfeld has a great deal of leeway to develop his service as long as the work is directly relevant to the goals and mission of the center. Because that is the case, it is his view that research reports are used and contribute to program development. Christenfeld's role is often one of assessing the feasibility of emerging program ideas. He is also impressed that Dr. Haveliwala has an excellent grasp of epidemiological research and can understand and evaluate data.

Research

Dr. James Smith heads an office of research. The office of research is less directly concerned with producing managerially relevant data. Research does have to be clinically relevant (for example, studies of tardive dyskinesia in age, sex, and diagnostic grouping). The office of research is charged with seeking outside funds for research. Some of its projects have received external support. Research emanating from Harlem Valley has been published in major professional journals and presented at national and international conferences. Dr. Smith now edits the *Harlem Valley Psychiatric Center Journal.*

Clinical research is conducted as a social obligation, but publishing research in major journals contributes to Harlem Valley's reputation as a center of excellence. An enhanced reputation is designed to make the facility attractive to middle-class patients who want to be treated in first-rate centers. Attracting middle-class patients is one of the center's goals. The director believes the viability of a public mental-health system depends on its serving more than the underclass the state hospital system has tended to serve in the past. Facilities with good reputations serving middle-class clients are more attractive to legislators, who in New York State have final authority in closing an institution. An institution with a good reputation is better able to attract highly qualified staff, thus improving patient care. Finally, the concept of a center of excellence has implications for staff pride in their own work and staff morale.

Review Committees

Harlem Valley has an extensive system of committees. The most recent revision of the By-laws of the Medical Staff lists 36 committees, lists their membership by role (for example, associate director, programs; chief of service, and medical-surgical chief of nursing) and contains a detailed charge for each committee. Many committees are concerned with planning or with operations, but many others are charged with reviewing or monitoring operations, including approving behavior-modification programs, reviewing psychiatric determinations of legal competency; incident review (untoward incidents, suicide, assault, accidents, and so on); patient abuse; and review of proposed research. All committees keep minutes of their meetings. These minutes are circulated and sent to the director's office where they are kept in a permanent file.

The Community Placement Review Committee is charged to evaluate and recommend what services should be provided to patients and what standards of quality and appropriateness should be sought in various levels of domiciliary facilities such as proprietary homes, and community residences and in community health institutions such as skilled-nursing facilities and health-related facilities. This committee, which has over twenty members, visits sites where patients have been placed in order to assess the quality of placement against Harlem Valley standards of quality and appropriateness. The committee is currently within the jurisdiction of the office of quality care to ensure appropriate service to patients living in settings outside the hospital.

The site visitors prepare a written report that goes back to the unit responsible for placement. These reports may be used as the basis for negotiating with the proprietor to correct deficiencies. They also contribute to clinical decisions concerning appropriate placement. These reports supplement data obtained from the program-evaluation unit that routinely tracks placements, recidivism, and follow-up visits to outpatient centers. A similar committee supervises family-care placements.

There is also a Program Review Committee. This committee's function is to: "Assess a program or a unit in terms of general administration, treatment program per se, staffing and education and training, through *on-site visits*, and make recommendations for further improvements and give positive reinforcement on positive features of this program." Each operational unit is subject to peer review. The peer-review results in a written report. Deficiencies that have been noted must be corrected. Members of the EC sit on both of these committees, and all committee reports are distributed to the director, who reads them. (He has a reputation among some staff for reading every piece of paper that anyone ever sends him. In fact, he sets aside two hours a day to read reports, memoranda, and the like. He does not read everything. His executive coordinator, Louise Hubbard, screens material for him, but she calls anything of significance to his attention.)

Inservice Education

While not technically part of the monitoring and evaluation system, Harlem Valley's extensive inservice educational program is part of the process that maintains a spirit of inquiry and growth. It is also part of the problem-solving process in that inservice education is used to train personnel to solve problems noted by the evaluation components, to develop personnel to serve new programs, or to improve the service that is currently being rendered.

Harlem Valley has developed a rather extensive inservice educational program. The organization of training has varied from time to time, but as with other Harlem Valley programs, the organizational position of each program was determined by a combination of interests and availability. There are essentially two wings, a professional education division that has been headed by Dr. Jerome Steiner, and a paraprofessional division headed by Jim Regan. Steiner is a psychiatrist in private practice and on the faculty of Columbia Medical School. He is a highly paid consultant in education and training to Harlem Valley. Regan is a psychologist who has served in several managerial roles in his time at Harlem Valley. Steiner, influential in professional organizations and well known in the psychiatric community, has taken the lead in developing training affiliations with medical schools. Regan has worked to develop contacts with community colleges, to bring courses to Harlem Valley, and to expedite the entry of staff into educational programs for their development.

Inservice education is also decentralized. Each unit defines its own needs.

If it does not have the resources to provide the training it needs, it calls on the central training unit for assistance. Many training projects emerge from identified needs within the unit, and sometimes program-evaluation data or special medical-care studies indicate the needs for specialized training. A single example will suffice. One unit began to show on its evaluation reports an increase in patient incidents involving assaults. Review of the problem revealed that staff had to rotate assignments, and many felt uncomfortable with acting-out patients. The unit decided it would be helpful if all staff, therapy aids, nurses, psychologists, social workers, and psychiatrists would receive some training in self-defense. The unit sent its request on to the central training unit. The central training office, along with a unit representative explored available programs. They found one that seemed appropriate. Scheduling for the program was worked out with the unit, and eventually all personnel assigned to that service took that training course.

The adequacy and relevancy of the training programs are monitored through a feedback system and through discussion in the EC. There is an education and training coordinator in each unit responsible for seeing that programs are developed, and responsible for reviewing the adequacy of programs to meet needs. Education and training is taken seriously because it provides continuing-education medical credits. Plans have been made to have the education and training coordinators maintain educational profiles on all employees, to monitor who is participating in educational programs, and to determine who might benefit from participation. These plans have not yet been put into full effect.

Although there is not a large centralized educational staff, a large number of people participate in the educational programs. Each employee is allotted approximately 10 percent of work time for educational purposes. The education and training chiefs call on staff in the various units to provide inservice education for each other, in their areas of expertise.

Under Steiner, professional education has enlarged to include the sponsorship of conferences open to the community at large. Harlem Valley is accredited to offer continuing medical-education credits, so these conferences can have attraction to a wide audience. Harlem Valley encourages its employees to attend the conferences, and sometimes will use its own funds to pay for their attendance. The conferences are sponsored through the New York State Mental Hygiene Research Foundation, or through another nonprofit corporation organized for that purpose. Sometimes the conferences turn a profit. The additional funds are then used to support projects that would be more difficult to support with state funds. The free-enterprise aspect of the system provides some motivation to make it work.

The development of educational affiliations with the New York Medical College Consortium has given Harlem Valley an important affiliation with an established psychiatric teaching institution. This affiliation is in fulfillment of a plan to have Harlem Valley become a major educational center. The plan is designed not only to ensure survival, by making the institution valuable to many community agencies, but also to improve services. The affiliations will allow New York Medical College residents to rotate through Harlem Valley. Harlem Valley can call on Medical School faculty for inservice education and for consultation. The affiliation is intended to further the objective of developing Harlem Valley's reputation as a psychiatric center so that its services become acceptable to the middle class.

Some Issues Raised by the Use of Resources for Evaluation, Research, Monitoring, and Education

Harlem Valley's program for evaluation, monitoring, research, and education has gone far beyond what one normally finds in a state facility directed toward service delivery. Harlem Valley seems intent on developing a multifaceted program in which a certain amount of its resources is directed toward other than direct service functions. The use of its resources in that way raises many questions. Some of these are matters of values while others relate to questions of what structures are necessary in order for a psychiatric center to provide the highest quality of modern services and to maintain a forward thrust in the sense that the center is continuously concerned with its own renewal.

Inservice Education

The training affiliation with New York Medical College provides the case in point. The affiliation involved extensive negotiations and indeed some selling on the part of Harlem Valley to make it attractive to the medical consortium. The expensive agreement provided funds to the medical consortium for its staff and residents. Staff and residents would spend only part of their time serving Harlem Valley patients or serving in consulting or teaching roles to Harlem Valley staff. The agreement did provide a prestigious affiliation for Harlem Valley. Whether it will provide an adequate return in terms of services or advantages in recruiting personnel remains to be seen. It appears to be true that a very large percentage of psychiatrists currently employed by the state system were first exposed to it as residents.

Some have criticized the agreement because of its high monetary cost. These critics argue that resources should have been expended to take care of immediate needs. They can point to a number of gaps in the community-support system and argue that filling those service gaps should have had higher priority than the educational affiliation. Moreover, these critics say the aim of reaching the middle class through excellent state facilities is chimerical, with resources thus wasted.

The counterargument states that the educational affiliation will improve services by improving chances of recruiting first-rate personnel and will provide top-notch inservice teaching for Harlem Valley personnel. Moreover, the concept of moving toward an educational and research center has motivating powers for current personnel, setting attractive targets for them to reach, and letting them feel they are part of an outstanding center. A center with an outstanding reputation also has greater chances of winning community support, and in the long run it may enhance the institution's chances for survival. Even if the agreement was expensive, supporters argue the affiliation could not have been attained in any other way, and it is sufficiently important for the long-range development of the center to be worthwhile. It remains to be seen whether the affiliation agreement will promote the ends its supporters envision for it.

Monitoring and Evaluation

The monitoring and evaluation systems go more directly to ensuring the quality of clinical services. Harlem Valley's feedback system is among the most elaborate we have seen in any service institution. Although norms for the distribution of clinical staff time into varied activities includes time for administration and for education, no one can actually say how much time goes into the various evaluative and monitoring devices. A few staff positions are devoted exclusively to these functions, but many personnel fill out forms, visit in the quality-assurance program, and participate in the many committee meetings, taking some time away from direct service. Is the amount of time spent in these several functions and activities a worthwhile expenditure of the center's resources?

On the negative side, staff say that some committee time is wasted, that not all take all committees seriously. Some complain that time is taken away from direct patient care and wonder whether the expenditure of staff time on monitoring actually improves services.

On the positive side, one can say that the monitoring and evaluating system is vital to the center's vitality since it is frequently a source through which problems are identified and corrective action initiated. The intensive review activity does lead to the maintainence of high standards. The review and evaluation data have been critical in the change process and in protecting the quality of care. The intensive review process probably resulted in slowing down the revolving door, and in avoiding the kind of dumping that makes newspaper headlines and sparks public investigations.

At first glance it seems as if a great deal of time is going into indirect service. However, we have no empirically valid standards to tell us how much staff time should go into which functions at different points in an organization's developmental history. Judged against the standard of most facilities that have wholly inadequate evaluation components, Harlem Valley's distribution of staff time in evaluation, education and research seems lavish. On the other hand, few state hospitals have transformed themselves the way Harlem Valley has. Its director asserts that most institutions use their resources inefficiently. He claims that by judicious reallocation of resources, the same budget and staff can be made to support many more varied activities. Given Harlem Valley's productivity, the director's assertion seems well worth considering.

9   A Viewpoint about Psychiatric Rehabilitation

Harlem Valley has transformed its program by reallocating its resources to different functions as its program developed. It used its program-evaluation system and its program and planning bodies to help determine how and when resources were to be reallocated and toward what ends. The process of reallocating resources was predicated not only on organizational considerations but also in relation to an understanding of the clinical problems of chronic patients discharged from psychiatric hospitals. Haveliwala had a thought-through plan for treating patients that guided decision making and that guided the establishment of priorities for new programs requiring the reallocation of resources.

In many states deinstitutionalization policy was based on the premise that resources necessary to maintain patients in local communities would be forthcoming as patients were relocated into community settings. In theory, to ensure that services were responsive to local need, local communities were expected to fund services. Since care of mental patients has largely been the responsibility of the state level of government, many expected that funds allocated to state services would be reallocated to local governments (Lamb and Edelson 1976). For various reasons the amount of money available was less than those interested in community-based programs had hoped. Many financially hard-pressed local governments are not pleased with the prospects of paying very much for services to mental patients. The development of appropriate locally funded services has lagged. Some observers believed that if patients were placed into communities, local government, faced with a problem, would respond by developing supportive services.

Although there are many complex factors associated with the phenomenon of dumping, so deplored by all (U.S. Senate Subcommittee on Long Term Care 1976), the assumption that resources would *follow* patients into the community was at least partly responsible. Resources did not follow patients into many communities. Rather, the support of released mental patients became enmeshed with the intricacies of the financial and political relationships among local governments, state governments, and the private, voluntary agencies.

Over and beyond considerations of financing and control, research indicates that released patients who return to hospitals do so within the first few months after release (Anthony 1979; Perry 1978). Patients cannot survive in the community unless supports are there and the patient is linked to those supports. Each person requires an appropriate place to live; a source of income; work; or training in preparation for work; recreational opportunities; appropriate psychosocial and medical care; and transportation either to bring the patients to services or to bring services to the patient. That is the essence of the concept of a community-support system. Either the psychiatric center has to provide such services, or it has to participate in coordinated-resource networks with a variety of community agencies. If no such network exists, the psychiatric center may need to work with local governmental authorities or with voluntary agencies to create such a network. Given this set of necessities, if the center were to fulfill its responsibilities to patients who were being placed into the community, it had to restructure its own operation. It had to take on new functions and deploy personnel differently.

Resources Should Precede the Patient into the Community

Recognizing the problems that emerged when patients were placed into communities without adequate support, the director of Harlem Valley built his program on the premise that *resources should precede patients into communities.* From his viewpoint, and the viewpoint of concerned staff, patients could not be simply abandoned. Rather, it was the center's duty to see that patients were linked to appropriate services; and if these did not exist, to provide them, or to help stimulate their development.

The assumption that almost all patients can survive in the community if appropriate facilities are available requires living and working environments, graded in the amount of independence each requires of the patient, and the amount of support each provides. Because the chronic patient released to the community was the hospital's first responsibility, the development of services targeted for that group took the highest priority.

Patients living in the community require a source of income. They need employment, welfare, or they must qualify for support as a disabled person. Relationships with county, state, and federal agencies and with employers had to be developed.

Appropriate living facilities had to be found or existing residential arrangements had to be modified so that patients could be located in them. It was not sufficient simply to find living spaces in the community. If patient interests were to be served, then they had to have access to graded living facilities in which degrees of supervision appropriate to the patient's needs at the time could be exercised. The therapeutic plan also called for the development of graded living arrangements so that patients could be moved from one setting to another as their conditions warranted. In fact, aspects of the program-evaluation system were directed toward monitoring the patients to help ensure that those who could would move on to more independent living situations. It became important to develop more family-care homes and to work with the family-care sponsors to see that patients moved on and new places were available. Unit Chief Jack Dominguez took the lead in this vital function. It was also necessary to develop good working relationships with skilled-nursing facilities, health-related facilities, and proprietary homes so that patients could be placed appropriately. For patients capable of more independent living, it was desirable to develop apartments. In some instances, a group of patients moved in with a staff member who helped them adapt to community living. In other instances, patients lived in small groups aiding each other, or they lived alone. When it became difficult to find landlords willing to rent to ex-patients, Harlem Valley developed an independent nonprofit corporation, Search for Change, that leased apartments in its name, and then subleased to discharged patients.

The director also believes that the most important single element in the treatment of chronic mental patients is the provision of real work or training. The development of graded work-related settings and programs also stood very high on his priority list.

Day care and assistance in managing activities in daily living, including recreation, were deemed important for other patients. If rehospitalization was to be avoided, crisis intervention including family members, care givers, and representatives of community agencies was essential. Transportation to bring patients to services and services to patients is a key element in developing and maintaining a community-support system. Most of these services were not available through existing outpatient clinics that offered psychotherapy and counseling or that provided periodic supervision of medication.

The director and his unit chiefs decided to develop the resources necessary to support patients in the community. If local communities did not provide the services or were unable or unwilling to develop them, then some personnel formerly devoted to inpatient care could be reassigned from their duties. While personnel experienced with chronic patients had some advantage in working with them, the skills and knowledge necessary to work in these new settings are different than those meaningful within the hospital setting. Not only was it necessary to make personnel available, it was also necessary to build a strong inservice educational component as part of the program. All these new activities could be developed only by reallocating resources.

Rehabilitation Begins in the Community

The director states that rehabilitation begins in the community. He refers this principle to research that shows that inhospital rehabilitative efforts and patient behavior in the hospital have little predictive value for behavioral adjustment in the community. Research supports the proposition that the nature of the patient's living and work situation, the support available, and the attitudes of the people who provided after-care and outpatient services determines recidivism more than patient diagnoses or manifestations of psychopathology (See Rappaport 1977, chapter 18). It follows from this premise that active, long-term treatment designed to cure psychopathology is less important than inhospital activities that prepare patients for community living.

Programming for newly admitted patients is directed toward the rapid reduction of symptoms and preparation for discharge. The utilization-review program, described previously, is used to ensure that each admission meets appropriate standards, that each patient has an appropriate treatment plan, and that the treatment plan is being followed, or if not successful, then revised. Programming for more chronic patients is also geared toward preparation for community placement whenever possible. Programming for the most regressed patients is aimed toward improving the patient's abilities in the activities of daily living. The goal is to move each person to the most independent living situation he or she is capable of tolerating.

The overall result of this treatment philosophy is that provision of resources for inpatient programming as for individual and group psychotherapy, or other elaborate recreational and rehabilitative programs has had low priority at Harlem Valley. Some of the problems attendant on this approach will be discussed.

Some staff report that some patients who were scheduled for discharge or release to community facilities were reluctant to leave the hospital. Some patients showed signs of anxiety in relation to an impending discharge and expressed reluctance to leave. Staff evidently took a very firm position about patients' leaving the hospital once discharge plans were made. Evidently, a patient's last-minute change of heart was generally not respected. Some argue that if patients had had sufficient preparation for discharge, they would have been less reluctant to leave the hospital.

The hospital did not commit any substantial proportion of its resources to developing programs designed to prepare patients to leave the hospital. The *Placement Service Policy and Procedure Manual* (revised September 1976) does have a release procedure (pp. 31–34) that includes contact with relatives; and a requirement that "Patient should see placement facility, be interviewed and approve the overall plan" (p. 31). Whenever a patient was to be placed out of the catchment area, the manual states that a letter requesting permission to place the resident must be sent to the director of the state psychiatric center servicing the area; that a copy of the letter must be sent to the regional director in Poughkeepsie; that an individual service plan had to be made in consultation with the receiving state psychiatric center; and that placement could not be made without approval of the receiving state psychiatric center. We must assume the written procedures were followed after September of 1976, but we do not know if they were prior to that date.

Patients and their families, as well as other psychiatric centers, were supposed to have been involved in the discharge-planning process. Clinical readiness for discharge was determined in unit staff conferences. Some programs such as family care were used to place high-risk patients with the understanding that many might return to the hospital. It was also understood that unsuccessful placements would be carefully reviewed so that they could be converted to successful placements on another occasion. The release-procedure manual is, however, silent on the question of how to handle patient anxiety or patient reluctance to accept discharge.

While there is little discussion of how patients were prepared for discharge, the placement manual does describe its AREA II Special Program for chronic patients. The goal of this service is to develop "placement readiness" through programs designed to improve communication skills, to teach activities of daily living including community-living skills, and to provide activities to prepare for the constructive use of leisure time. At the time the manual was written, 58 patients were in this program. Evidently some inhospital preparation for discharge went on, but it is not clear how much of it went on during the period when patients were being released at a rapid rate.

Harlem Valley's director justifies his decision not to commit any substantial resources to programs designed to prepare patients to leave the hospital on the basis that research has shown that such preparatory effort does not predict adjustment to the community, that rehabilitation takes place in the community. The director's view is completely compatible with the conclusion reached by Anthony et al. (1972) and Anthony (1979), in their extensive literature review of studies of psychiatric rehabilitation and the similar conclusion reached by Perry (1978) in his review of follow-up studies since 1972.

Clinical lore has it that symptoms sometimes recrudesce at the point of termination of treatment and that such a regression is no necessary reason to change termination plans. It is also true that critics of large state-hospital programs have charged that one of the failings of such programs is their tendency to foster dependency in their patients. If dependency was fostered, anxiety about becoming more independent is completely understandable. It is clinically sound to respond to such separation anxiety with the firm expectation that the patient can tolerate the separation.

Some authorities (for example, Braginsky, Braginsky, and Ring 1969) assert that chronic patients have a vested interest in living in hospitals and do not find their conditions at all aversive. As far back as 1889, the New York State Commission on Lunacy recognized that some paupers sought out the comforts of institutional living. The commission asserted that early commitment laws were designed, in part, to keep paupers from signing themselves into hospitals. Professional employees in the Veterans Administration mental-hospital system recognized a type of patient informally called a "snow bird," a patient who traveled south for the winter, and north for the summer, signing himself into appropriate hospitals at both ends, and sometimes along the way. Towbin (1969) reported an experiment in self-government for chronic patients. While

the self-government program resulted in considerable improvement in participating patients, few made any movement toward discharge until the staff took
an active role and insisted on it. Evidently some number of patients do need
strong encouragement to leave a mental hospital.

While no one could condone actions such as those reported by the U.S.
Senate Committee on Long Term Care (1976) describing patients unycere-
moniously placed on buses and deposited in nursing homes, without any preparation or follow up, no one seems to claim that was what Harlem Valley did.
Harlem Valley staff claim that patients and their families often visited nursing
homes or family-care homes prior to their placement. Obviously, not all families
of all patients visited the homes and approved them. Some staff told of white
families who protested at the placement of the ex-patient with a black family
in a black neighborhood. If so, it is obvious that either such a family was not
fully apprised of the placement or that their wishes were not always respected.
We do not know that all patients visited their new homes and approved them.
However, many staff did visit the homes. Unit chiefs encouraged staff opposed
to the deinstitutionalization thrust to make such visits especially to proprietory
homes, skilled-nursing facilities, and family-care sites. Presumably they would
not have agreed to placement in undesirable facilities.

It is not clear that staff judgment should necessarily supercede patient
judgment in such matters, but evidently some effort was made to see that placements were suitable. It is possible that a less rapid pace of deinstitutionalization
might have left more time or careful preparation of patients. If it was sensible
to discharge clients to other community facilities, it is not clear that more
elaborate preparatory programs would have significantly reduced patient anxiety
about discharge, nor that it would have improved their chances for adjusting
favorably in the community. Authorities are in general agreement that post-
hospital care is the major factor in reducing readmission rates (see Anthony et al.
1972; Anthony 1979; Rappaport 1977, chapter IX; Perry 1978). The director's
strategy in allocating resources to the development of outpatient care rather
than inhospital preparation for release is justifiable in terms of contemporary
knowledge.

10 Creative Administration and the Reallocation of Resources

The new approach required that resources be reallocated from existing services to community-based services since new resources were not to be forthcoming. The reallocation of resources required creativity and educated-risk taking on an administrative level. In this section, we will describe something of the administrative maneuvers used in finding and reallocating resources.

"Where There's a Will . . . "

In the very first EC meeting, the director asked each unit chief to provide him with a list of buildings in their service that could be consolidated with others or closed. At the time there were about 45 wards with about 50 patients in each ward. Each ward had about 25 staff. In order to free some personnel to develop community-based services before patients were discharged, the director hit upon the tactic of closing down two of the wards and redistributing patients to the remaining wards. If patients were distributed equally to all wards, then each would have received two to three additional people to serve. The director knew that any overcrowding would be temporary because patients would be placed into appropriate community settings at a rapid rate. If any untoward incidents resulted from this practice, staff opposed to deinstitutionalization have not specified them.

It is not always the staff from the closed services who were sent out to develop community-based services, but the approach freed up people who could be used in those roles. Unit chiefs found volunteers willing to work outside. As the first group developed the community-based resources and as placements were made rapidly, more staff could be used to develop additional outpatient resources without taking away from inpatient care.

No one was required to work in an outpatient setting. Unit chiefs asked for volunteers, or they traded with each other to get people who were interested, willing to work in the community, and with the skills and personal styles to function with uncertainty. Initially, most outpatient employees came from the Harlem Valley Hospital. The center developed a huge transportation system, at first using employees' personal cars and later center vans. At a later date when programs were established and as personnel lines opened up, people from the communities in which center outpatient facilities were located were hired. Those who participated in the early, exciting days remember them fondly as a time when all were working hard and were sharing successes and failures. Many good friendships were formed during those exciting days, friendships that persist.

Creative Administration

Much depended on the director's ability to reallocate resources to new services and to the variety of staff functions the elaborate system requires. In a psychiatric center, the primary resources are personnel, or "items," in personnel language. Budget and personnel are allocated to centers annually on the basis of formulas relating the number of personnel, the distribution of types of personnel, and total number of dollars to the number of patients served. Because the budgeting process is geared toward inpatient care, the formulas weight the number of inhospital patients very heavily in determining the number of personnel necessary to care for them.

At Harlem Valley the director and the EC took advantage of budgetary rules by reducing the inpatient census rapidly. Items (personnel) designated for inpatient care could be reclassified, and people hired to do other jobs. (This strategy was carefully thought through, and depended on the cooperation and skills of the then-personnel officer, and later deputy director for administration, Wendy Acrish.) The center did not lose proportionately more items for personnel in subsequent years. According to New York State Mental Hygiene Department budgetary standards, it had been understaffed to begin with. Moreover, personnel assigned to outpatient care tried to develop large case loads to justify their continuation.

The skills necessary to function in staff roles and in outpatient settings are not necessarily the same as those required in inpatient settings. It was necessary to reassign and reclassify positions in order to hire people with the appropriate skills. Budgeting rules do provide some flexibility in that one can reclassify positions. Thus one can take an empty therapy-aid line, and create a position for an MSW Social Worker, assuming there is room for a professional line within the allocated distribution of types of positions. As long as total budgeted dollars are not exceeded, nor the total lines exceeded, items can be reclassified with the approval of the Mental Hygiene Department Personnel Officer, the appropriate division within civil service, and the Division of Budget.

Obtaining approval for reclassification of positions, writing job descriptions, and presenting the credentials of people to show that civil-service requirements have been met is a technical matter requiring knowledge and experience. In reclassifying positions, Harlem Valley administrators were always very careful to observe the letter of the law and to document each case appropriately. Failure to do so can create enduring, time-consuming problems. Deputy Director for Administration Wendy Acrish, a career administrator within the New York system, was justifiably proud of her excellent reputation. Because she had years of experience with the system and had excellent working relationships with people in the appropriate offices in Albany, Harlem Valley requests for personnel reclassifications were rarely turned down.

Harlem Valley administrators occasionally found creative solutions to personnel problems. Once when a professional line necessary at Harlem Valley was not available, Ms. Acrish used her extensive network of relationships with personnel officers in other institutions to "trade" items. She carried two lower-salaried staff for the other institution on her payroll and assigned them to detatched service to the second institution. The second institution in turn hired the professional person Harlem Valley wanted and assigned that person on detached service to Harlem Valley. This maneuver is a good example of creative bending of the rules because it is not permitted to shift personnel items from the budget of one institution to another. Harlem Valley administrators were fully aware of the possibilities and were perfectly willing to take educated risks to promote programmatic ends.

A Budgetary Process

Each year the director has to prepare a budget for the center and defend the budget in relation to the program. The process of defending a budget is designed to keep the budget honest, to ferret out fat in it, and to try to ensure by means of budgetary control that objectives are being attained. He has a face-to-face conference with a budget officer from the New York State Department of Mental Hygiene and defends his program. The director is said to be very effective in defending his budgets because he has a thorough mastery of the budgeting process and an intuitive grasp of figures. The detailed program-evaluation reports are put to excellent use in the budgetary conference. Haveliwala can defend his budget because he has the figures, and he knows them very well.

Harlem Valley has adopted an internal version of a budget process. It has been different each year, but basically it requires that each unit chief submit a budget for personnel items. These are projected against current workload, the anticipated decline in patient census, and the anticipated development of new programs with an increasing outpatient load. One year these budgets were reviewed in an EC session, and allocations were made on the basis of that review. The session led to some complaints about slave trading in secret sessions. In another year, an all-day workshop was held in which program submissions were discussed openly in the presence not only of members of the EC but also other department heads as well.

According to some observers, there was only a small change in the allocations from submissions, suggesting a prearrangement. However, other experienced observers felt that the open process had kept unit chiefs and department heads honest since they could not fool each other about their needs. Their submissions reflected hard thought about their needs. Whatever the open process contributed, it certainly made all aware of the problems in reallocating resources and probably provided excellent training for assuming executive responsibility.

Allocations of personnel and other resources during the formal budget process is not the only method. Many project ideas emerge informally or as a result of emerging opportunities. Haveliwala believes that it is useful to start several projects concurrently because not all come to fruition. Moreover, it is not possible to predict precisely when a program would be ready for implementation. Aware that he could count on a certain amount of attrition (retirements, people resigning), he engaged in a game that could be called "budget roulette." More personnel were tentatively allocated for given projects than there were items on hand or in sight. An overrun could result in a loss of budget for the following year and create problems in staffing services. A budget overrun could also harm the director's and deputy director's reputation with upper-echelon managers in Albany.

The director, desirous of moving the center forward and aware that loss of momentum could impede change, pressed forward. State budgeting practices encourage overspending because they often come through with year-end bonuses because there are unexpended funds. Haveliwala was willing to take risks by spending to the limit and assuming it would work out. He initiated new projects or encouraged others with ideas. Sometimes more than one person was encouraged to look into the same project or into different versions of the same project. For many projects there was an implied promise of resources. Where the director drove the system forward, encouraging program staff not to think of monetary restraints, it was the role of his deputy director administration, Wendy Acrish, to call budgetary realities to his attention and to find creative ways of meeting programmatic needs with available funding. She and the business manager, Margaret Grant, worked effectively to find the resources, even though they also had to work against the pressures of other staff who were encouraged to proceed without worrying about where money would come from. In order to develop outpatient facilities, it was necessary to lease space. It required the business administrators to develop standards for such space and to clear arrangements through the state bureaucracy. There was also considerable effort in finding the resources to improve the physical environment of the wards. Such improvements required a great deal of innovative management and juggling of resources in order to support the effort to develop new outpatient space while improving existing inpatient space.

Once Harlem Valley decided to establish community residences to increase placements, it was the job of the deputy director, administration, and the business office to find a way to support their development. Mrs. Grant developed a budget request, with the assistance of the regional office and the Division of the Budget, which was identified as a certificate "to pay on a revolving fund basis for the establishment of resettlement apartments for discharged patients." This was a unique use of an existing account, the patient interest account, which was never before tapped to provide security money, deposits for utilities, rent advances, furniture, or furnishings. The use of this fund, in this fashion, enabled Harlem Valley to send patients out into prepared residences and at the same time to offer landlords the kinds of assurances that they needed in order to be willing to rent out apartments to former mental patients.

Patients' interest funds were also used in a second unique way. Actual cash was given to clients to use specifically for trips accompanied by staff into the community where they would eventually resettle. The purpose of the trips would range from getting comfortable in the community to job hunting.

In addition to developing special budget certificates for the use of patient interest accounts, the business officer and the office of the deputy director, administration, found ways to better utilize regular state budget funds, particularly to meet the needs of humanization. Regular on-going meetings were held by the purchasing departments with clinical staff so that together they could design an appropriate living environment. The results of working together were coordinated purchases that met patient's physical as well as esthetic needs. The wards now show evidence of serious efforts at personalization. Bedspreads, sheets, and drapes often match. Lamps and night tables are individualized but still coordinated with the rest of the room. Much of the furniture in the large day halls is conducive to small-group conversation yet still safe and functional. In most hospitals purchasing is done in large lots without consulting ward staff. The result frequently leaves much to be desired, functionally and aesthetically.

In order to assist in getting patients back into the community, the community-store funds were used in another special legal account, that was set up specifically to support volunteers in taking patients into their homes and into restaurants. In many programs even if the volunteers are willing, the costs present a financial hardship to many. Funds from the community-store and patient interest accounts were set aside so that volunteers could take patients to recreational and rehabilitative activities in the community. The funds were designated for recreational and rehabilitative activities for the patients and the volunteer that accompanied them.

Regular state budget funds for utilities were also used by the business office to pay for utilities in community spaces that were donated. During the period of expansion into community programs, the state institution as such was not allowed to pay rents. It was difficult enough to get an agency to donate space, and virtually impossible to ask them to also pay high utility costs on this space. At the time Harlem Valley could pay the utility cost for donated space. This practice is no longer permitted, but at the time it was critical in acquiring appropriate community space for programs.

Largely through Mrs. Grant's efforts and rapport with her support staff, stored or discarded furniture was converted into attractive pieces to enhance the environment. For example, old night-stand tables were cut down, rebuilt, and made into planters. A chair that was in need of upholstering was painted and re-covered to coordinate with a patient's room to add an additional touch of homi-ness. Support staff spent many hours constructing partitions out of lumber or devising ways to divide large areas into smaller, more private, areas. None of this was above and beyond their job descriptions, but had they not been cooperative, it would have been necessary for the institution to submit a capital construction budget request to purchase equipment or to have it done by outside contractors.

The tactic of starting many projects created some internal problems. Some-times projects would reach a stage of readiness for implementation, and re-sources were not available for it. Under those circumstances the individual who developed the project would be asked to put it aside. If the individual had a lot of time and libido invested in the project, disappointment followed. Sometimes promises had been made to others outside, and a certain amount of backtracking and undoing followed. Unit chiefs say that once a firm commitment had been made, the director always delivered for them.

Obviously, not all projects worked out, nor could all be staffed. When he makes a decision, Haveliwala is always careful to explain his reasons. His explana-tions helped to ease disappointment and to maintain morale. Most of his staff are convinced that his decisions are made on the basis of program considerations and not personal favoritism. They accept their disappointment as a temporary hazard of the game. Most executives feel they can come back with the project at another time or that another of their projects will receive support.

In defense of the process, it should be said that active risk taking frequently resulted in new program development. Since the center was fighting for its life, the rapid development of community-based programs and innovative programs was necessary to ensure its future support. The director seemed impatient to get things moving, but given its circumstances, perhaps Harlem Valley did not have the time to move slowly.

The Effect on Inpatient Care

Reallocated resources came primarily from inpatient services and reflected the decline in patient census. Personnel to staff outpatient settings came from re-sources originally allocated to inpatient services. Similarly some of the resources that went into direct patient services such as evaluation and monitoring and in-service education, were released for reallocation in relation to the declining in-patient census. However, the problem is not that simple. There is not a linear relationship between declining patient census and declining personnel needs. The plant and grounds need to be maintained. Food services, laundry, purchasing, and other administrative functions have to go on. Inpatients require twenty-four-hour coverage. All these services and functions require their own numbers of people even if the patient census is reduced. Since Harlem Valley's policy was to deemphasize institutional care and to concentrate on the development of out-patient services and the community-support system, it is reasonable to inquire about the effect of the reallocation of resources on inpatient care.

There is a dispute about whether in-patient services have been helped or harmed. The Director and many of his Unit Chiefs are convinced that there is a great deal of inefficiency in inpatient services and that appropriate supervision can result in better patient care, with the number of personnel available or even with fewer. The director also argues that inpatient staff ratios have actually been improved as a result of change. His executives argue that the hospital generally is better off for the elaborate development of programming and evaluative devices.

From an objective viewpoint the quality of inpatient care has probably improved over time. Well-qualified professionals have been hired, and medical-psychiatric care improved. Untoward incidents and instances of patient abuse are relatively infrequent. These are monitored and investigated throroughly. The Joint Commission on the Accreditation of Hospitals has renewed Harlem Valley's accreditation, although it did recommend that inpatient programming be increased to some extent (August 1977). Overall, the charge that inpatient care has declined cannot be sustained.

Many of those working with chronic patients in the hospital do not feel quite the same way about the effects of reallocating resources. They feel their workloads have increased since they now have a higher density of difficult-to-manage patients. Recreational programs are absent on weekends and evenings. Personnel are spread thin on night shifts. They also seem to feel their services are less important in the total scheme of things and fear that further reductions in the inpatient census will result in a loss of their jobs. They note that professionals have replaced paraprofessionals. Many do not wish to relocate. The elaborate development of community-based programs is not in their interest. Line personnel also assert that patient care in the community is poor and that patients do not receive the benefits of recreational programs, good food, and medical care available in the hospital.

Whatever else the reallocation of resources has accomplished, it is clear that not all interests have been served. It is possible that more attention to the needs and views of inpatient staff may help to ease some of the morale problems. The director is aware that the spirit of the program has not yet permeated all levels of the organization, and he is concerned; however, until now, other matters have had priority.

Relations with the Union

The union plays an important role in constraining changes by enforcing contract provisions that define the conditions of work for its members and by acting to preserve jobs for its members. The union is also concerned wth improved patient care, recognizing that good patient care serves the interests of its members as well. The union may well have its disagreements with deinstitutionalization policies. The ability of any director to reallocate resources depends in part on union cooperation. Under some circumstances, the union may well be able to complicate changes by resort to the grievance process or by bringing indirect pressure through its ability to use political power with elected officials.

Harlem Valley has had relatively little difficulty with its union during the change process, even though the contract is the same as in other state institutions. There are several reasons for the relatively peaceful labor-management relationships. There is no tradition of militant unionism at Harlem Valley. In years past the relationship between the director and staff was best characterized as paternalistic. Employees had job security, and the custodial orientation of the hospital was relatively undemanding. Moreover employees were like family. People lived together on the grounds, worked together, were married to each other, were friends, relatives, and neighbors. Apparently, situations that might have led to disciplinary action or to grievances were usually resolved informally.

Recall the hospital was fighting for its life. Employees, fearing the hospital would close down, offered no active resistance to anything that looked as if it could save the center. Many were apparently willing to give the new methods a try. Leadership at the unit level seems to have been very effective as well. When changes were instituted, employees were consulted. Efforts were made to take employee wishes into account and to provide incentives for change. No one was forced to take on outpatient duties, but rather volunteers were sought. Management made an effort to make the new working conditions attractive for employees. Travel time was granted, employees were given generous allowances for use of their own automobiles, and a flexible time arrangement was worked out that gave some employees a four-day week.

During the early phases of the change in 1975 and 1976, employees who were displeased did have an option. Because of the Willowbrook Consent Decree (1973 and 1975), a nearby institution, the Wassaic State School for the mentally retarded, expanded its staff. Moreover, to relieve overcrowding at Wassaic itself, many of its residents were moved to Harlem Valley buildings under Wassaic's mangement. A number of staff were able to take positions with Wassaic without loss of pay or seniority and without having to change residence. In some instances former Harlem Valley employees benefited by obtaining positions at higher grades.

The director claims he made an effort. Active union members believe that the union was consulted only when trouble was anticipated or when specific contract issues were involved. The union is not represented on the EC, for instance.

At present the union and others report that morale among the paraprofessional staff is low. The union leadership concedes that no one has been fired, but the union is also aware that losses have been the greatest in the paraprofessional ranks. The union believes that changes have led to an increased workload for ward-level inpatient staff. The various monitoring devices are not experienced by ward-level staff as providing information useful to them but rather as checking up on them. Ward-level staff complain that they feel mistrusted by upper-level staff and that some recent events have exacerbated that problem. The union also believes that management shows little interest in informal resolution of problems with employees and warns that if the trend continues, formal grievances will be filed more often.

The union complaints are consistent with the director's recognition that the spirit of the institution has least affected ward-level and paraprofessional employees. Given that the life situation, culture, and motivating forces of the different groups are different, it appears to be a distinct problem to try to develop a process that meets the needs of all levels. At Harlem Valley, history, circumstances, and efforts to accommodate minimized labor-management conflict. In another institution, the factors could well be different. A change agent would have to assess their significance in context.

The Bureaucracy's View of Creative Administration

Harlem Valley has pursued an independent course. Although its general objective of reducing the inpatient census while providing outpatient care and follow-up services is in keeping with New York State Mental Hygiene Department policies, its methods for reallocating resources and for producing change depart considerably from the general practice. Since Harlem Valley is part of a large bureaucracy, the bureaucracy's view of its methods are of interest.

We have already indicated that Harlem Valley used made-up titles, had people working out of job description, and had developed a number of departments that do not exist in other institutions. Harlem Valley found the resources to develop its programs by taking skillful advantage of the budgetary process. In addition, each of its community services developed an advisory body. Some members of the advisory bodies have used personal and political influence in favor of the center's programs. The center has developed an unusual agency, Search for Change, a nonprofit corporation that subleases apartments to patients released to the community. In pursuit of its educational programs, it has developed an affiliation with a medical center requiring the use of a substantial amount of center funds to pay salaries for medical-school faculty and for fellows. Its educational program included the sponsorship of large conferences featuring nationally known but expensive speakers, for which fees were charged to participants. Arrangements have been made with the Mental Hygiene Department Research Foundation to handle these funds outside of the hospital's regular budget. Similar separate "pockets" have been developed to handle other funds that come to the hospital. These funds have been used to pay for trips to conferences and to cover similar expenses and pet projects that would not have been readily fundable through the regular budget.

In developing these activities, all legal requirements have been met scrupulously. Audits of the various funds have confirmed that all expenditures were for appropriate purposes and were appropriately documented. These arrangements are familiar. Anyone who has worked in a research university that receives funds from a variety of sources will recognize them. Various accounts are handled separately for bookkeeping purposes, but funds from the several accounts are used for providing programmatic flexibility. The arrangements, while not unusual in some settings, are unusual in a state agency. From that viewpoint they properly create concern among officials in the state Mental Health Office, in the Department of the Budget, and in the Civil Service System.

Some of Harlem Valley's activities have resulted in conflict with county mental-health authorities, and with some voluntary, private agencies, and with other state psychiatric centers. Harlem Valley placed its clients outside of its own catchment area and indeed outside of state limits. These activities have led to charges of dumping. These conflicts have reached the commissioner of mental health. The director, in pursuit of the center's objectives, has also made public statements and involved himself in legitimate political action, but sometimes he adopted an independent position that may have been contrary to the State Department of Mental Health's wishes. His statements and independent actions have been viewed by some as bold and by others as abrasive.

The director believes that the state system should provide excellent service. In pursuit of that objective, he has insisted on traveling "first class," housing some of his outpatient units in excellent locations, and in spacious, well-decorated facilities. Some believe the private, professional mental-health community is unused to seeing a vigorous, highly professional state service that is overtly and covertly critical of them. Others believe it is unseemly for a state agency to aspire to first-class status when such status involves expensive facilities.

Harlem Valley also has developed an active public-relations division. It has announced its accomplishments to the human-services community, but sometimes its bold announcements have led others to denigrate its accomplishments or to concentrate on the program's inadequacies.

All these factors result in rumblings in the small world that is the state system, and rumblings attract official and unofficial attention. As far as we can determine, officialdom maintains an attitude of respect for accomplishment, a deep interest in how change was accomplished, and natural skepticism that all is as advertised. Distance lends enchantment, but it can also contribute to a vague uneasiness on the part of those who necessarily view any new and unfamiliar development from the perspective of people responsible for a larger system.

The director has made distinctive efforts to confront issues related to the larger system of which his center is a part. He and his administrators have been scrupulously careful to develop new projects within administrative guidelines and within the law. The director is always very careful to know his position, and to understand what he can and cannot do. He seeks advice before he acts. He has also employed his deputy director for administration and his business manager as control and as supports in the sense of having them find creative ways to use the fiscal resources available to the center. In acting, all have been very careful to observe protocol and process.

He has been careful to let officials in the State Mental Hygiene Department know what he is doing. He invited the regional director to attend any or all meetings of his EC and has regularly mailed EC meeting minutes to that official. His activities have been very public, and he has called attention to what he is doing. In many instances, he invited critics to participate in center programs, and in the course of doing so, has won respect and support from several. He has cooperated with state projects, offering his facilities for the development of a level-of-care survey, for example. He has cooperated with some training programs originating at the state level.

He has a good understanding of the value of what he has accomplished, is willing to bargain hard for what he wants, and is willing to maintain an independent stance, even in relation to the state department. His independent stance may not necessarily win friends and influence people, but it does require that others take him into account. It may be that a bureaucracy has to learn to live with its system buckers if it is to encourage and respect differences that contribute to revitalization.

11 Embedding Programs in the Community

As soon as one thinks of community-based treatment and community support systems, one must consider the elaborate structure of governmental and private services that exist in the community and the attitudes and feelings of citizens toward having formerly hospitalized patients in their midst. Change goes on in a dynamic social context that includes tensions among county government, state government, and private voluntary agencies.

The history of mental hospitals in the United States reveals the problems very well. In colonial days the mentally ill were cared for either by their own families or were placed with the poor, the chronically dependent, and the immoral in almshouses or in jails (Deutsch 1949). A few private hospitals were built. State facilities developed when it bacame clear that local government and private philanthropy and organized charities were unable to assume the burden of care for so many.

When in the early and mid-nineteenth century states accepted responsibility for providing mental hospitals, the political system immediately had its effects upon care. There were state-local government conflicts of financing from the earliest days. In Massachusetts, for example, local governments were assessed for the care of their residents sent to the state hospital. Local communities therefore kept their more manageable patients and sent only the more violent and difficult ones. The state hospitals, receiving more difficult patients, quickly filled with chronic patients, taxing their meager treatment resources further. We mention this history to remind readers that the political conflicts described in this section are built into the American system, have been with us for a long time, and are likely to be with us in the future (Bockoven 1972; Caplan 1969; Gish 1972; Grob 1966; 1973; Rothman 1971).

Consistent with Anglo-American traditions in social welfare dating back to the Elizabethan Poor Laws of 1601, responsibility for welfare is placed first on the family; second, on private voluntary agencies; third, on local communities; and fourth, on central government (that is, state and federal levels). Agencies of central government have absorbed more of the responsibility for funding social welfare as local and private resources have proved inadequate for the tasks, but the ideals persist.

New York State's policy in the field of mental health is to encourage the provision of community-based services through local and state shared funding (Mental Hygiene Laws, chapter 251, as amended to 14 April 1978). The state Department of Mental Hygiene accepts the mission of providing institutional care. With the contemporary change toward community-based services and a decline in the census of institutions, pressure on local government to provide outpatient services has been increasing. The state tried to make it financially attractive for local government to provide outpatient services, through a formula that reimbursed counties that funded selected services. The mental-hygiene law acknowledged the role of the private sector by permitting local government to contract with private agencies for services reimbursable by the state. The mental-hygiene law explicitly encourages cooperation among local, private, and state providers, but the mechanisms to ensure cooperation leave a great deal to be desired.

Several factors interfered with policies designed to ensure cooperation and coordination among state, local, and private service providers.

First, many county governments, hard pressed to meet their expenses and faced with taxpayer resistance, are reluctant to extend their financial commitments, even though the extended commitment brings state dollars to their county.

Second, citizens in many local communities were not receptive to having mental patients relocated among them. Therefore county governments felt an underlying political pressure against extending services that would bring and help mental patients in their communities.

Third, existing voluntary agencies may not be equipped to provide the services necessary to maintain former mental patients in the community. Many voluntary, private agencies provide specialized services to selected clientele. For example, a family-service agency may provide couples counseling and family therapy to those willing to come into an office and talk with a social worker or other psychotherapist. Such services may be inappropriate for a former mental patient placed in a group-living situation in a YWCA, who needs assistance in job placement and in coping with other activities in daily living. Many agencies feel they are not prepared to provide services to different groups of clientele. Moreover, they argue that there is an overwhelming demand for their services.

Fourth, deinstitutionalization policy creates a conflict for employees of the state system. To the degree that funds go to support community-based agencies, to that degree the economic and career interests of state employees are adversely affected. State employees' opportunities for stable employment and advancement are better if community-based services are provided by the state directly rather than through a transfer of funds from state Department of Mental Hygiene to county Departments of Mental Health.

Fifth, the state, county, and voluntary systems of care function in an elaborate and interlocking political structure. The state Department of Mental Hygiene is responsible to the governor and to the state legislature. The governor and state legislators are elected officials who balance the political and financial feasibility of any policy with an assessment of what is necessary to provide services for the people of the state. At the county level, commissioners or directors of mental health are responsible to elected county executives and a county legislature or to citizen boards.

Working within the constraints of funds and programs that are reimbursable with state funds, some county commissioners negotiate contracts with private, voluntary agencies to provide services. Others provide them under county auspices. The voluntary agencies receive part of their funds from quasi-private sources such as the United Fund. They have boards composed of influential citizens who not only oversee the agencies but who also advocate for them. The voluntary agencies, their professional directors and staffs, and their board members constitute a political bloc. They have interests in pursuing their own service missions and in advocating for funds to be allocated through sources that will best serve their purposes. Similarly, the county commissioners wish to have as much control as possible over the provision of services in their counties. The state Mental Hygiene Department, which provides services to the institutionalized population, has its own needs. If the state perceives that county governments are not providing the services necessary to support patients in the community, then it must allow the state psychiatric center to provide some of the necessary services. Otherwise the department can be accused of callously dumping patients on local communities.

Sixth, deinstitutionalization requires services that the state Mental Hygiene Department cannot provide. Patients' need for income cuts across other governmental lines. Welfare, or Medicaid reimbursement for care involve state and county Departments of Social Service. When the applicant is eligible for disability payments under the federal Supplemental Security Income program, the federal Social Security Administration is involved.

Many patients are placed in skilled-nursing homes or in board-and-care homes operated under private auspices. Many of these placements are funded by Medicaid, a joint state and federal program. The proprietors of the facilities have an economic stake in reimbursement rates and in the services they are required to supply to earn their rates. The governmental services agencies are responsible to see that humane standards of service are met and to control costs. The proprietors of the facilities also constitute a political block with common interests.

The interests of Mental Hygiene and Social Service departments are in conflict. To the degree that patients are placed in the community and in proprietary homes, fiscal responsibility is shifted to the social-service budget, but the social-service responsibility to provide services is unclear. Even if they wished to do so, social-service departments do not have the resources to provide what patients need.

Human services are quite fragmented. The Department of Mental Hygiene is now divided into three offices: mental health; alcohol and substance abuse; and mental retardation, each with its own commissioner. The three commissioners are urged in the legislation creating them to consult with each other and to cooperate, but each office has its own views. There is an office for services to the aged under a totally separate administrative structure. While there may be valid reasons for the separations, the fragmentation when added to the problems of working with local government and the private sector results in difficulty in providing continuous and coordinated services.

When Harlem Valley embarked on its program of placing its patients in the community and when it insisted that its patients would have appropriate services, the complex of governmental and private agencies became a vital part of its task environment. If its programs were to survive, much less thrive, they had to be related to the community context. Harlem Valley had a strategy for extending its programs into the context.

The Community Context

Harlem Valley's service area is large, extending into three counties, diverse in its socioeconomic characteristics and in the character of its community organizations. The approach to each community has to take into account the nature of the community, the nature of existing services, and the nature of citizen involvement in the service structure.

Eastern Dutchess County in which it is located is not a part of its formal catchment area. Many of the small local communities in this rural area depend on Harlem Valley economically. Harlem Valley patients are placed in residences in Eastern Dutchess communities, in family care, or in proprietary homes. Mobile teams follow these patients, or outpatient care is provided for them. Putnam County is growing very rapidly, but it is relatively undeveloped as far as a local service network is concerned. The county's consciousness of its needs for a service network is just beginning to be raised.

Westchester County, on the other hand, is densely populated, has an elaborate network of voluntary service, including some for chronic patients, and has a tradition of active citizen participation in the service network. Westchester County varies in its socioeconomic characteristics from the wealthiest of suburbs to poor inner cities with minority populations and enclaves of working and lower-middle-class white ethnic groups. Westchester County has its own hospitals, including a county psychiatric facility, Grasslands, which treats on a short-term basis, and refers long-term clients to Harlem Valley. Part of Westchester County is also serviced by another state facility, Rockland Psychiatric Center. Because geographic boundaries are not the same as functional boundaries, some ambiguities exist about who is to do what to whom and where.

Harlem Valley had service and organizational objectives in moving its programs into the surrounding communities. First, it had a responsibility to provide for its patients who had been placed in community residences. It had to see that the residences were adequate and were adequately supported with consultation and crisis services. Second, it had a responsibility to link its clients to other community supports. Its clients would require day care and other rehabilitation services in addition to supervision of medication. Third, if it was to work to prevent hospitalization, it would have to relate to community members in addition to former hospital patients who were living in the community again.

Harlem Valley also had organizational objectives. Although the director full well realized that Harlem Valley might be closed down as its census dropped, he was concerned about developing viable, community-based services that would be of value to its former patients and to the surrounding communities. Moreover, from the point of view of the morale of Harlem Valley personnel, it was important that they believe their efforts could contribute to organizational survival, if not as an inpatient institution, then as an organization providing a range of valuable services.

It operated with the important assumption that adequate mental-health programming could best be provided by the state. Recent experience had shown that local governments in many communities could not provide sufficient funds nor sufficiently stable funds to provide continuity of care. Harlem Valley adopted a strategy of providing its own supportive services as much as it could, by developing outpatient facilities.

In pursuit of the objective of developing programs of value to local communities, its first programs were for populations not served by existing service agencies. As a part of that strategy, it also used its resources (jobs, funds for leases, positions on community advisory boards providing some influence and status) to win the support of community members. It used these services as bases from which it could expand its offerings to its patients and to the community.

Barriers to Cooperation

The problem of entering a community to provide services is very different, depending on the characteristics of the local community, and depending on the amount and kind of services that exist. The situation may even be different in different sections of the same county where urban-rural differences may have resulted in very different kinds of private services. As a general rule, conflict was encountered when the psychiatric center's definition of the necessary services and the local government's definition differed or competed.

Westchester County, the most densely populated of the counties in Harlem Valley's catchment area, had an elaborate network of private and public services. These were concentrated in the southern and central portions of the county. There were fewer service providers in the northern section of the county. Westchester had created local advisory councils consisting of representatives of its contract service agencies in the three regions. At the time Harlem Valley entered the Westchester community, in 1974 and 1975, county agencies were feeling the pinch of the economic recession and cutbacks. County agencies were not in a position to develop new services for the deinstitutionalized because county governments were not supportive of new programming during this period. The local council system, particularly in the southern and central districts was described as cumbersome and as dedicated to seeing that existing agencies continued to receive funding for their programs.

The local agencies were unable to develop new programming, even if they wished to do so, and it is questionable whether many were interested in providing extensive services to the chronic population. Some of the local agencies had serious reservations about the state facility's developing programming in their areas. The reasons were complex. Some felt that the state agencies would provide inferior services and pointed to the fact that state agencies could staff outpatient services with less well-qualified people than would local private agencies, which had to meet state certification standards. State facilities did not need to meet the same standards. Some felt that the state would begin encroaching on traditional private-sector-service territory particularly in an area in which there were already many services. Others indicated they felt some twinges of professional jealousy when they realized the state had funds to reallocate to outpatient services, but they had none. Some felt that Harlem Valley's offers of shared personnel showed how rich the state was in resources, compared to the pinched conditions in local communities, and these attitudes led to some resentment of Harlem Valley people.

Observers point out there was very little conflict in Northern Westchester. There, few service agencies functioned, and county mental-health authorities recognized the need for day-care services. It was much easier to come to agreement with Harlem Valley people about what was to be done in that section of the county because both groups had the same service priorities. Apparently, in central Westchester, Harlem Valley personnel began not by providing direct services but by providing the equivalent of case-management services, linking former Harlem Valley clients with local services and supports. According to Westchester authorities, that set of functions led to much less conflict since all agreed the services were necessary and useful. It was after Harlem Valley developed more elaborate outpatient services and began serving other populations that conflict developed between state and county facilities.

The situation in Putnam County was again different. The mental-health agency in Putnam was valiantly struggling with a huge overload and huge waiting lists. Local legislators, however, were uninterested in developing more locally sponsored services. Harlem Valley's services were needed in the area. However, mental-health personnel in Putnam experienced the Harlem Valley approach to them as the city slicker telling the country bumpkins what to do. Putnam mental-health-service providers felt that their intent and desire to develop a range of services, although constrained by budgetary limits, were not recognized by Harlem Valley personnel, at least not initially.

Later as Harlem Valley services developed, Putnam mental-health personnel expressed some concern that Harlem Valley personnel were not consulting them sufficiently about plans for residences for mental patients. Putnam personnel felt they would bear the brunt of community resentment for Harlem Valley actions in establishing residences for mental patients. They were also concerned because they had few facilities for emergency hospitalization of mental patients whom they felt needed institutional care. They experienced Harlem Valley controls over hospitalization as unduly restrictive. Over the years Putnam County and Harlem Valley mental-health personnel learned to work together and are now making a distinct effort to cooperate and to coordinate services.

There were efforts to develop shared staffing programs in a number of areas. Harlem Valley offered to make personnel available to county-sponsored facilities in order to help develop appropriate outpatient facilities for former Harlem Valley clients. These arrangements never worked out. Some say the offers were not made in such a fashion that they could be carried out. Others say county agencies were not willing to work together with state employees. Whatever the professional prejudices, or whatever the machiavellian motivations attributed by either side to the other, the fact remains that shared staffing arrangements present realistic administrative difficulties under the best of circumstances. Salary scales, holiday schedules, supervisory structures, staff meetings calling people away from the office, reporting forms and the like are different between county and state. There are difficulties in determining who receives credit for reimbursement purposes, for providing services to patients. In some instances patients have been double billed because of such arrangements. Most recently auditors for the state raised questions about whether state contributions to shared staffing should be considered a state contribution in kind as part of the state's share of funds to be reimbursed to counties. If that happened, counties could lose cash they expected to receive. On all these administrative grounds, cooperative staffing arrangements seem difficult at best. If in addition there are feelings of competition and mistrust of intentions, it is easy to see why the fond hopes for cooperation between state and local governments, as expressed in legislation, have rarely come to pass. There are built-in reasons for the problems, and these cannot be readily attributed to any given individual's personal style.

Providing Services in the Community

In one of its communities, the Harlem Valley unit chief found that existing agencies could not service Harlem Valley clients adequately, and for internal financial and political reasons could not expand sufficiently to accept the increasing load of deinstitutionalized clients. A highly influential professional leader was opposed to the entry of new services. Given the existing complex of programs, Harlem Valley concentrated its efforts on developing geriatric services. There were no geriatric services in the community, and many of the patients who were released were elderly. Geriatric services were welcomed by existing service agencies. and Harlem Valley personnel were accepted as specialists in the area.

Space for a geriatric day-care center was leased from a church in a black neighborhood. The church, once assured that its members could also use the center's services, supported the center. The church also welcomed the rental it received. Its minister was encouraged to participate as a religious counselor. As staff positions became available, community members were hired on a full-time basis, replacing the white workers from the hospital. By then the hospital staff, supervised by Nurse Janice Ek (one of the managers whose skills transcend their professional training), had developed an active program, including the provision of daily transportation to and from the center for clients they felt needed to attend. As the program developed, Ms. Ek began consulting with other agencies about cases they had involving elderly clients, and she began offering the center's services to them as well. The exchange of resources enhanced the position of the day-care center in that community, developed political support for Harlem Valley, and gave it a legitimate base in the community. From that base, Harlem Valley was able to participate more directly in the deliberations of existing community councils, and it became an integral part of the local service network.

By participating in deliberations of local councils, and by consulting with representatives of local government, and the service network, a Harlem Valley unit chief determined that an alcohol-treatment program was necessary and would win support in that community. Although Harlem Valley had some reluctance to enter the area of providing outpatient alcoholism services, the possibilities of winning the cooperation of local authorities was persuasive. Harlem Valley did develop an alcoholism-treatment unit whose functions were later taken over by another agency following the reorganization of the state Department of Mental Hygiene.

Robert Tannenbaum, the Harlem Valley unit chief in Northern Westchester, worked closely with Zelda Domashek, a representative of the Westchester County Mental Health Board to develop a group of service providers concerned with after-care services in northern Westchester. The coordinating group worked closely with the Northern Westchester Mental Health Council and existing coordinating councils. Harlem Valley also used its field staff to cooperate with other agencies in helping them to achieve their objectives. When one agency was interested in developing an ambulatory health center under a regional medical-care grant, a Harlem Valley social worker was assigned to the project to provide it with support in mental health.

Harlem Valley found that it was difficult to continue to place those of its chronic patients who came from there in New York City. Moreover, for many who no longer had family and friends, a New York City placement made no sense. Eastern Dutchess County was a relatively depressed area with many homeowners who were happy to accept suitably screened patients into family care or into a boarding-home arrangement. Harlem Valley began by extending its family-care program in Eastern Dutchess County. Jack Dominguez, another of the talented Harlem Valley executives who participated in many of its programs, was prominent in this effort as well. The Dutchess County commissioner of mental hygiene was not opposed to the extension of family-care services in that part of the county partly because there were no services there and partly because patients in family care are still considered psychiatric-center patients and are not the county's responsibility. The psychiatric center that served Eastern Dutchess County as part of its catchment area had no plans for additional services in that part of the county. Meanwhile the New York State Mental Hygiene Department had recently established regional offices to aid in the deinstitutionalization process. The development of community-based services was consistent with its mission there. Given that coalition of interests, Harlem Valley was able to negotiate for an extension of its services into Eastern Dutchess County, even though that geographic district was not formally within its catchment area. Jack Dominguez organized a group of family-care sponsors to help solve problems, negotiate terms, and to help recruit other sponsors.

As long as Harlem Valley programs were developed in service areas lacking in the particular community and were developed cooperatively with local government and local providers, little conflict emerged, and the services were welcomed. However, in areas more densely populated with service providers, it was more difficult to find areas of cooperation. Some existing agencies provided services suitable for chronic clients, but the variety of services was limited. Nonetheless, influential service providers, either fearful of competition, desirous of maintaining control over a territory, or having serious questions about the professional adequacy of the credentials of state-hospital employees, declared opposition to Harlem Valley programs.

Harlem Valley, feeling that existing programs were inadequate to meet its patients needs, moved to provide services for its patients even in well-serviced sections of the community. Its first effort was to offer to develop jointly staffed programs, or to contract for services with the established agency. The existing agency rejected the offer. Strategically, the offer would have established Harlem Valley as a service provider either way, and as noted previously, there are realistic administrative difficulties in jointly staffed programs. The rejection of the offer allowed Harlem Valley to continue to pursue its own course.

It was not without allies in its effort to establish itself as a service provider. The service network was by no means unified in its opposition to Harlem Valley. For example, an evaluation that was sponsored by a local citizens board, of an existing local service for chronic patients found that it was inadequate to serve its purposes. The negative evaluation weakened the opposition to Harlem Valley's participation in that community. Harlem Valley executives moved to take advantage of the situation by forming a coalition of interests with those who had past differences with the way the local mental-health council functioned. The negative evaluation supported the need for new services, but to consolidate its political position in the community, Harlem Valley hired, as a paid consultant to their developing community-based operation, a person who had been influential in the evaluation process. Harlem Valley also found it could form coalitions of interest with some agency directors in influencing the allocation of local funds to attain mutually acceptable service objectives.

Unable to arrive at fully satisfactory agreements with local-government and local-service networks, Harlem Valley decided to use its own resources to establish multiple-purpose outpatient centers. The director was aware of his powers and willing to use them. He could reallocate resources under his control (for example, staff and funds to lease space) to the development of outpatient services. With the advice and assistance of his deputy director, administration, and his business officer, he was able to find creative ways to maintain budgetary flexibility in order to fulfill plans or even to take advantage of fortuitous circumstances. In one instance a team of eight highly qualified professionals, experienced in working with state-hospital patients, indicated their willingness to move as a group from another hospital in which all were employed. Because he had budgetary flexibility, he hired the entire group and established a respected professional team in the community as a fait accompli.

This action was not without its later complications. In order to develop a large enough case load to justify the size of the team, the group did a great deal of outreach, sometimes offering services in direct competition with those offered by existing agencies. Political opposition, combined with the financial incentive to the county under unified-services-funding principles to monitor state services, led to continuing conflict about the amount of service rendered and the cost per unit of service provided by Harlem Valley staff compared to other agencies. Differences in the definition of a unit of service used by county agencies and by Harlem Valley did little to clarify the issues but did contribute much to continuing conflict.

Haveliwala participated personally in many meetings with community agencies. He tended to assert strong positions and made no bones about his willingness to move unilaterally if he and representatives of other community agencies could not arrive at satisfactory agreements. Although he asserted strong positions, and although his forthright manner was considered abrasive by some, observers are in general agreement that he usually made a clear and rational case for his position, as well as a forceful one. He was aware of the power he had and was willing to use it. For example, he was able to reallocate resources under his control to establish the services he felt were needed. However, he did need some degree of assent from the existing community structures. Because he participated actively and persistently, he was able to persuade many of the correctness of his position. Moreover, he had some bargaining leverage. Under the existing mental-health legislation, the community mental-health board required his assent to unifed-service plans submitted to the state for approval for reimbursement. When Harlem Valley deemed the community mental-health board's plans inadequate, with the assistance of state mental-hygiene officials, he was able to block their plans.

It is difficult to determine all the factors involved in these conflict-laden negotiations. Some Harlem Valley staff feel there was adamant opposition in

the Westchester professional community to their presence and that no negotiation would have succeeded. Other observers feel that the director's approach
to negotiation was highly abrasive, leaving a strong residue of ill feeling. Still
others believe that the community was not ready to deal with many of the
difficult mental-health problems and that only a vigorous encounter with an
outside force was sufficient to unfreeze the situation. Some of the Harlem
Valley unit chiefs found the director's role as a "heavy" helpful in the sense that
they were able to adopt more conciliatory postures with their counterparts in
other service agencies. Not all the conflict persisted. One member of the then-
existing community mental-health board who was once an adversary moved
closer to Harlem Valley's position and in fact became a member of its Board of
Visitors.

Why did the director insist that he would go ahead with or without the
cooperation of local officials and professionals? Some believe that his plan for
the center's development required that outpatient services be provided under
Harlem Valley auspices. These critics believe that a softer stance, which might
have led to continuing negotiation, and the development of less debilitating
political conflict, would have reduced the need for Harlem Valley's services in
the community. The director believed he had to do whatever he could to provide
community-based services to support patients living in the community and to
prevent hospitalizations. Protracted negotiations would have delayed the development of services for patients who urgently needed them.

In order to maintain a sufficient case load, Harlem Valley outpatient units
offered their services to populations served by other agencies. There were simply
not enough chronic clients to be found. Chronic clients are difficult to track
and to keep in a service system. Some die. Some leave the area. Some refuse
further services and make their own way. A few violate the law and go to jail.
Needs-assessment techniques have not been very accurate in showing just how
much service of what kind is necessary for chronic clients. Some local providers,
not only in Harlem Valley's catchment area but elsewhere as well, have been
asking, where do all the patients go?

Haveliwala was aware that he may have been acting, if not in opposition to,
then not in keeping with such policy as existed to support locally funded and
locally operated, community-based services. Aware that such locally funded
services were not forthcoming, to implement the state's deinstitutionalization
policy without "dumping," he had to see to it that services were provided. He
calculated, shrewdly and accurately, that once he had established the necessary
services, the Department of Mental Hygiene would support his actions. Indeed,
the department did not reduce his outpatient budget in subsequent years beyond
the expected decline in budget with the decline in the inpatient census. All concerned recognized that Harlem Valley's programs did provide necessary patient
care not provided by other agencies.

Community Advisory Boards

Each outpatient center developed a community advisory board. Eventually, a local advisory board for the hospital itself, in addition to the board of visitors, was created to help improve relationships with the center's immediately surrounding communities. Advisory boards fulfilled an ideal of community participation, helped to develop support for Harlem Valley, and its members brought resources for the center's programs.

Unit chiefs strived to develop advisory boards with independent minded, active citizens. Not only did Haveliwala believe in his programs but he also believed that strong people, convinced of program quality, would actively support the effort to provide needed services. Moreover, strong individuals with many contacts in the service network, could help, not only by offering advice but by using their political and social connections to provide significant assistance for Harlem Valley programs and patients.

Strong individuals would insist on expressing their own views. Sometimes community board members would adopt positions different from ones Harlem Valley's director and executives would have preferred. Under those circumstances Harlem Valley's director and executives engaged in a mutually educational dialogue with their board members. Sometimes the board member would understand the center's position and sometimes the center would see reasons for moving differently.

In some communities there is a mental-health power structure consisting of active influential citizens who frequently serve on several agency boards and on committees, task forces, and study commissions. Some are well-to-do people with close personal ties to the local business community and to local politicians. They have ready, informal access to people like themselves who serve on other boards and are invaluable when they work for social agencies. (Dahl 1961; Graziano 1969; Heller and Monahan 1977; Hunter 1963).

Board members do not receive tangible benefits for their participation. They may on occasion influence contracts, leases, or employment in the agency. They may also occasionally assist personal friends in obtaining agency services. In general, the rewards are psychological. One obtains satisfaction in fulfilling an ideal of service, in becoming expert in agency functioning, in exercising influence, or in sharing in the excitement of struggle and accomplishment. Occasionally such individuals receive personal recognition in the form of awards.

Harlem Valley has made good use of the advisory-board structure. It appointed strong individuals to its community boards, carefully selected them from among influential people in the community, and nurtured their interests by giving them real responsibilities. Its unit chiefs meet regularly with their advisory boards. They keep them fully informed and call on them for assistance with given projects. Whenever the center's EC meets in one of its decentralized locations, a representative of the advisory board is invited to attend to participate in the discussion and to confer with the director. One staff member has been assigned the task of relating to advisory-board members, to maintain their interest, and to recruit new advisory-board members as necessary.

Advisory-board members have served a number of purposes. Because they have affiliations with other agencies, they can serve to introduce Harlem Valley staff and programs to other agency directors. Because some are recognized as people with influence, they are able to talk to public officials to help expedite programs. For example, an advisory-board member was instrumental in obtaining Park Department cooperation for a garden project. In another instance, board members used their own network of acquaintances to help increase attendance at a fund-raising affair. An influential citizen took it upon herself to place a call directly to an official in the New York State Mental Hygiene Department to inquire about the status of a lease for program space. The center director could not have made the call without going through channels, but the advisory-board member could exercise direct influence. Advisory-board members have been encouraged to communicate with local legislators and to testify at legislative hearings.

Harlem Valley has introduced a reward structure for its board members as well. It paid expenses for some to attend statewide conferences. More important, it rewarded some active board members by submitting their names to the governor for appointment to the center's board of visitors. Several who have been appointed to the board of visitors on the director's recommendation served as community advisory-board members. The possibility of being recommended for such an appointment adds to the motivation of some to serve.

The approach has led to the development of a vigorous board of visitors who can advocate for the center and who at the same time can be strong in advocating for patients and for the community. The center's board of visitors now includes among others an individual who owns a local radio station; several prominent public-spirited citizens long active in community affairs; and an individual who was the center's adversary when he was a member of his community's mental-health board. These individuals continue to represent their own positions and have not always agreed with the director's views. The director believes the center is better served by a strong active board than by one that simply rubber stamps his decisions. Even though the independent board has adopted positions that led to conflict with the director, the director and board have a mutually respectful relationship and see each other as working toward common goals.

Problems in Community Relations

Although the center had been very careful in its relationships with distant communities, two incidents underscored that the center also had to concern itself with its immediately surrounding community. In one of these a group of local residents protested the use of a building on the hospital grounds as a half-way house. The building was directly across the street from their homes. Although the residents were familiar with patients, and several worked on the hospital grounds, they were adamant in their opposition to the open facility. The center's executives were surprised at the amount of feeling that local residents showed. They attributed it both to the resentment that many felt about the deinstitutionalization policy and to the fact that the present center's leadership did not socialize with local community leaders as their predecessors had.

In a second incident, a patient was struck by a truck on the public highway that passes through the center. The accident stimulated further demands that the hospital follow a locked-door policy. The director met with local citizens and explained the hospital's program and its obligations to its patients. He was forthright in stating that he could not accede to their demands, but he did acknowledge a problem. The center worked with the citizens to develop a committee to work on the problem. Eventually the committee influenced highway traffic authorities to reduce the speed limit in the vicinity of the institution.

These two incidents and protests that some neighborhoods in nearby communities were being saturated with family-care and boarding homes for ex-patients, led the hospital to be more responsive to its local community. The center then formed an advisory body for the hospital itself, composed of influential citizens including many local town officials. This group is just beginning to function, and it is too early to tell what effect it will have on improving community relations.

The selection of influential citizens for advisory boards has been generally effective. However, some feel that the patient-consumer should also be represented on advisory bodies. There have been some inconclusive experiments in that direction. The patient must be selected carefully. In one instance a patient with too many obvious symptoms proved to be disconcerting to other advisory-board members. In another instance hospital staff took umbrage at the presence of a former patient on a committee. Some members of the hospital staff believed the former patient was highly prejudiced against them, and they resented some of that individual's actions and attitudes.

Not all efforts to develop community boards have been equally successful. In some communities it has been difficult to find enough interested people to sustain significant effort. Sometimes a board will fail because of internal conflicts. Harlem Valley continues to have faith in the principle despite some failures.

The existence of strong community boards has created some problems for the center's management. Unit chiefs may develop close personal ties to board members, some of whom are very influential. The relationship of the unit chief to the board can provide the unit chief with an independent power base. The unit may develop programs that are not fully in keeping with center priorities.

Sometimes the board members unit chiefs recruit are opposed to the center's direction. Their influence may limit the expansion of programs that bring more chronic patients into that community. The problems are those that arise when strong-minded, vigorous people pursue their own ideas. On balance, the advantages seem to outweigh the disadvantages, but the problems are mentioned to dispel any myth that community participation is conflict-free.

Volunteer Services

Harlem Valley has an extensive volunteer program, inpatients' services being coordinated by Camille Giuditta and outpatients' services by Alifiyah Haveliwala. Volunteers offer tutoring or companionship. Others act as sponsors for former patients in the community. Still others operate a store that provides patients with inexpensive clothing; the store also earns some money to support the volunteer program.

The hospital has been careful to integrate its volunteers into its work. The inpatient director of volunteers has a number of assistants who supervise volunteers, provide consultation for them, arrange for their assignments, and generally clear the way for volunteers to function in the institution.

The center feels that its volunteer program serves several purposes. First, it extends the hospital budget. Volunteers provide many activities and services the hospital would otherwise be unable to afford. Second, the volunteer program helps to educate the community about the hospital's work. Third, the volunteer program increases the center's value to its local community. Many of the volunteer programs are tied in with high school and college educational programs. The hospital gains volunteers but in turn provides an educational laboratory for its community.

The volunteer program is very well organized. A written contract spells out the volunteer's commitment and the hospital's responsibilities. The volunteer participates in an orientation session and receives further training and supervision from the five hospital staff assigned to work with them. Volunteers participate in team meetings whenever possible. Every six months the volunteer receives a written evaluation from the supervisor, and each one is asked to submit a written critique of the program as well.

Public Relations

Harlem Valley employs a full-time professional public-relations specialist. The incumbent, Muriel Shepherd, is an experienced journalist. Her task, in addition to writing brochures for the hospital, is to develop active relationships with the local community to increase acceptance of mental-health services and of patients placed in the community. Her office has conducted a series of mental-health-information days, directed toward the lay and professional communities. She assists local reporters in developing human-interest stories favorable to the center and its programs. Rather than responding passively, the public-relations office tries to develop good working relationships with local press, radio, and television reporters.

Rehabilitation Programs

Harlem Valley participates in Cooperative Industries, a consortium of seven organizations that sponsors 60 workshops and does $1,000,000 in business. The consortium pools its resources to enable each member to share the benefits of centralized contract procurement, reduced competition among them, and limitations on machinery, transportation, equipment, and storage space. Cooperative Industries is an unincorporated association that works through cooperation. Member workshops share the costs of its operation. Cooperative Industries solicits contracts throughout the entire Northeast. Once a new contract is obtained, workshop directors decide which workshop and which clients are most suitable for the job. One agency assumes primary responsibility and then subcontracts work to the other participating agencies. The workshops not only share contracts but they also share equipment so that machinery does not sit idle. The arrangement has worked effectively and provided steady work for clients in the system.

The program was organized by Harlem Valley Psychiatric Center, the Hudson River Psychiatric Center, and the Wassaic Developmental Center. Later the Middletown Psychiatric Center was added and also three private workshops, Dutchess County Association for Retarded Children, Putnam Industries, and Rehabilitation Programs, Inc. The consortium has proved to be of great benefit to patients as well as its members. Because of the interlocking nature of the workshop arrangements, patients can move easily between the state and private systems as they are placed in the community. Harlem Valley patients, for example, may be placed in a community-supported workshop and later when discharged work in that same workshop. The transition is eased for the patient.

Former patients have an incentive to work. Income from sheltered-workshop employment in nontaxable and does not count as income to be subtracted from welfare or supplemental security income grants. Patients have some motivation to earn more money. Patient funds are handled through the hospital's business office. Contracts are negotiated on the basis of minimum-wage hourly rates. Patients are employed on a piece-work basis. Most do not earn the minimum wage, but some earn far over it. The workshop retains a small profit on its contracts to pay for its participation in the consortium and for other expenses.

Harlem Valley has developed a transitional employment system. The system has programs graded in their demands for work skills and independent responsibility. Harlem Valley identifies thirteen different types of vocational opportunities ranging from a prevocational training center designed to resocialize clients to a program of placement of clients in competitive jobs or training positions in private industry. Harlem Valley operates its own sheltered workshop at Wingdale but in addition has ten satellite shops. Some of the satellite shops are located in community residences (that is, adult homes) that house Harlem Valley patients. Harlem Valley places its clients in existing workshops and provides psychiatric support or, when appropriate, shared staffing arrangements are worked out. It also relates to the state Office of Vocational Rehabilitation and seeks appropriate training funds for its clients.

The varied vocational settings allow supervisors to adopt a more therapeutic attitude toward clientele. Formerly if a patient did not fit in, the patient was returned to the ward. Now, with psychiatric consultation and with varied settings available, staff work to try to adapt the client to the work situation. In-service education has also resulted in a better understanding of psychiatric symptomatology and a more sympathetic approach to patients. A former patient who relates well to patients has been hired to supervise one shop. Harlem Valley is currently negotiating to obtain a regular state job for him.

Because a patient's work situation is so intimately tied to his living situation, responsibility for housing is also in the same organizational division as responsibility for work. Both are under the direction of Dave Sorenson, who is also responsible for the community support system program and its extensions.

Search for Change is another example of how Harlem Valley programs are organically linked with community programs to provide advantages to both and to provide smooth transitions and graded opportunities for center patients.

Search for Change

Search for Change is a nonprofit corporation developed by Harlem Valley to help it solve a problem in finding suitable living quarters for patients placed into the community. Even though some patients have stable sources of income, many landlords are reluctant to rent fearing former patients would be irresponsible. To meet that problem, Harlem Valley organized Search for Change. Search for Change leases apartments and then sublets them to Harlem Valley patients. Search for Change agrees to be responsible for the rent and for damage to the property. In turn, Search for Change collects rents from patients, retaining a management fee to sustain its operations.

The corporation was organized by Harlem Valley. Its president is Sam Gordon, a member of the center's board of visitors and a member of one of the community advisory bodies as well. A retired businessman with investments in real estate, Mr. Gordon is very active in the social-welfare community, serving on many boards and committees. Mr. Gordon is very knowledgeable about real estate and has many personal friends among landlords and builders. It was through his influence that Search for Change was able to lease a number of choice apartments in brand-new high-rise buildings.

Search for Change has adopted the strategy of seeking scattered sites for their apartments because they do not wish to create resistance by making their entry into the community visible. Moreover, scattered sites help to prevent the creation of "psychiatric ghettoes." It also obtains apartments because zoning regulations and other laws limit the uses of single-family residential properties. An early experience with extended negotiations and public hearings around the use of houses in residential neighborhoods led to a preference for apartments.

Search for Change is a good example of a creative response to a problem that involved the community. When it was first organized, a Harlem Valley staff member was assigned to work with the fledgling corporation. Seed money for the Search for Change apartments was provided from interest on patient accounts, funds that can be used for patient benefits. Furniture and household goods for the apartments were from stored equipment formerly used in staff housing. The deputy director, administration, and the business manager were instrumental in finding these resources. Once it was organized and had funds coming in, Search for Change hired the Harlem Valley staff member as its full time director. Search for Change now is independent of the center, although it works for the center's patients. It is now considering building some facilities of its own under federal programs. It is also expanding its operations into other communities than the few in which it originally leased apartments.

Skilled-Nursing Facilities and Board-and-Care Homes

Harlem Valley embarked on its deinstitutionalization program at a propitious moment. Federal and state programs had encouraged the expansion of privately owned skilled-nursing facilities. Proprietors were eager to have patients to fill their beds. Harlem Valley took advantage of this situation by working aggressively with proprietors on the one side and with the Harlem Valley staff on the other to prepare patients for discharge to appropriate facilities.

While many institutions placed patients in nursing homes and in other domiciliaries, Harlem Valley went about it very systematically. Moreover, they followed their patients into the community. During the very first EC meeting in July of 1974, Dr. Haveliwala announced that he had spoken with the owner of a newly built adult home who was willing to accept Harlem Valley patients. The proprietor was willing to integrate the patients with other clients who would use the home as a general residence. The agreement permitted Harlem Valley to screen all patients for placement. The home would provide the maintainance and housekeeping staff while the center would provide some staff to assist in managing patients during the adjustment period. Harlem Valley also agreed to provide back-up psychiatric services and to work with the home to develop vocational and recreational programs. This initial venture with the Crestview Manor is still in operation and has provided something of a model for such services.

Harlem Valley's deinstitutionalization effort depended on finding sufficient beds so that geriatric and other chronic clientele could be placed rapidly. Harlem Valley executives, competing as they were for placements, worked closely with workers who provided the liaison between Harlem Valley, the nursing homes, and the state and county Departments of Social Services, which paid the bills. While a number of people did similar work and contributed to the development of Harlem Valley's placement system (for example, John Civitello and Betty Wright), Rosalie Lichtenstein, who did placements for the geriatric service, a service that had a long-standing reputation for excellence, eventually took primary responsibility for nursing-home placements.

An important step was to develop a detailed knowledge of the procedures of the several county social-service departments and relationships with people in those departments. She learned how to do the paperwork in order to expedite placement and become familiar with case workers and supervisors. Many departmental personnel were invited to Harlem Valley to participate in meetings or picnics. A good part of her work was with the New York City Welfare Department because a large number of the patients had originally come from New York City. The knowledge Harlem Valley placement workers developed was not only useful in doing the paperwork. It was also helpful in working with proprietors of nursing homes. Using their knowledge of social-service rules and procedures, Harlem Valley workers helped the proprietors with paperwork in order that they might qualify for the highest rates New York State would allow them to receive for patient care. The proprietors appreciated the help they received and welcomed Harlem Valley placements.

Unit staff made contacts with patients' families and brought the patients to the homes for trial visits. Most important, the unit chiefs were willing to commit Harlem Valley mobile teams to work with the patient and the nursing home's staff as needed. Those visits not only provided support for the patient but they also provided regular review of each home's conditions. If the conditions were inadequate, they could negotiate with the owner to correct them. Sometimes Harlem Valley provided staff around the clock; then as the patients settled in and the home's staff got used to working with them, Harlem Valley staff would slowly withdraw. Eventually a consultant would visit at intervals but was on call. The support made Harlem Valley patients more attractive to the proprietors. In some instances, proprietors were cooperative in providing programs as long as they needed more residents. Harlem Valley staff visited as long as they were placing patients. However, in a few homes, services deteriorated after the homes were filled. Some observers felt that some proprietors may not have acted in good faith. Others felt that Harlem Valley teams visited distant homes primarily when they were placing new patients and that the distance made it difficult to maintain regular contact. In any event, once a large home filled with clients, it was difficult to act to change the situation if it was a poor one.

It was not only the patient who had to be prepared for placement. Many of the inhospital staff had reservations about the readiness of patients for discharge. Each patient had to have a packet of completed forms that contained information relevant to a determination of the patient's eligibility for placement and for funding. In order to complete the forms, the staff had to review the patient and recommend discharge. Working within a medical model, staff would point to diagnoses or describe patient behavior in the language of symptoms, for example, hallucinates or disoriented. A language emphasizing illness created barriers to community placement. Unit chiefs favored describing patient's actions in behavioral terms, for example, sometimes talks to himself, or forgetful but able to care for self. (Court decisions which state that a patient may not be held involuntarily unless the patient is dangerous to self or others, imply behavioral, rather than illness criteria. The behavioral emphasis is in keeping with legal requirements.)

Those staff who believed in the benefits of community placements would read every record before every clinical meeting. They would carefully cross-examine other staff who were resistant to community placement. If a patient was characterized as "assaultive," team leaders or the unit chief would carefully call attention to the date of the last incident report and go into a detailed description of the events. It might turn out that two years earlier, the patient, very angry over a frustrating event, had cursed loudly and knocked over some furniture, but had calmed down readily when staff talked over the problems with him.

When focused on a careful behavioral description of each event, staff would often find it difficult to defend the use of psychopathological terms. The more benign descriptive language improved the patient's chances for being considered eligible for community placement, from the viewpoint of the social-service department and from the viewpoint of the owner of the proprietary home.

A great deal of paperwork had to be completed before each patient could be placed. Each county had its own forms and its own requirements. Since Harlem Valley was placing patients in homes in several counties, and indeed in Connecticut and Massachusetts as well, the paperwork was complex. Based on consultations with each social-service department, Harlem Valley executives developed a model packet for each one, including all the necessary forms and the requirements for eligibility. The model packets were made available on each unit. Unit chiefs then established production standards for each social worker assigned to their unit so that the paperwork was ready as the patients were ready.

To help assure staff that patients were being placed responsibly, unit chiefs had many of them accompany the placement workers as they visited the 37 facilities in which patients were being placed. Seeing new, clean, brightly decorated living quarters (many of the homes were new and just opening), some, but by no means all, staff were reassured that what they were doing would indeed better patients' lives. If a facility were not adequate, that message would soon filter back, and staff would be more resistant to placement there. After it started, Placement Review Committee reports served the same function as staff visits had earlier.

In 1973 and 1974, social-service departments did not seem to be overly concerned about the numbers of people they were supporting, nor was there much indication of community resistance to placements. Although county social-service departments had final responsibility for placement, de facto responsibility was in the hands of the clinical teams at the hospitals. The social-service departments would generally approve placements that the hospital's staff approved. Homes were opening rapidly, and spaces were there to be filled. In placing across state lines, Harlem Valley worked out informal agreements with the state's Department of Mental Hygiene that in the event rehospitalization was necessary, the patient would be returned to New York. Given good working relationships and given that Harlem Valley was careful to honor its agreements to provide assistance as necessary, placements were expedited. In fact, after homes were filled and spaces became tighter, proprietors would inform Harlem Valley of openings.

The situation has since changed. Departments of social services, painfully aware of rising costs, have acted more vigorously to control eligibility and to limit reimbursement rates. Political scandals that emerged around some of these operations (not necessarily ones that involved Harlem Valley) have made them less accessible and to some extent less attractive as alternatives than they once were.

A new problem emerged once patients were placed out. The center became dependent on the homes and lost some leverage with them. There is great potential for abuse in this situation, especially in view of the director's pressure to place. At Harlem Valley the independent Placement Review Committee was one control against abuses. A second was the norm staff established that they themselves would not accept inferior placement. The problem was more difficult to control at distant homes, especially if the proprietor was not eager to maintain expensive services that seemed to have been promised when they first took patients in. In general, Harlem Valley personnel succeeded, but it is true that some placements were less than fully desirable.

The example indicates how careful staff work, close administrative control, and the search for alternatives mutually beneficial to the center and to community agencies resulted in rapid but careful placement. Once again, we see the center integrated its resources with the needs of agencies in the community in order to accomplish the center's aims.

12 Issues, Problems, and Policies

In this final chapter we will discuss several related issues. The first is a consideration of leadership style in an attempt to separate out issues that are idiosyncratic to this particular leader from those that arise because of the way the leader has defined his role and used his discretionary powers. The second is a consideration of the relative balance between a human-service organization's use of its resources for its own benefit, as against the use of resources for client benefit. In the course of considering the balance, we will touch on further policy questions concerning the role of a psychiatric center director. Finally, we will consider issues related to the diffusion of innovation. If Harlem Valley succeeded in changing itself in the best interests of its patients, then its methods repay study. This section will consider some factors that affect a dispassionate appraisal of Harlem Valley's accomplishments.

Leadership Style

The leader of any organization is an object of special attention because of the position itself and the special privileges and perquisites of office. Leaders wield power that can affect people's lives. Moreover, many leaders exhibit personal qualities that stimulate emotions and motivate people to effort. The leader of a changing organization is very likely to be a controversial figure because the change effort may require others to alter their ways of thinking and believing as well as their activities. Power, status, financial rewards, and job satisfactions are all affected by change efforts.

Students of leadership (for example, Hollander 1978) assert that the single most important characteristic of a successful leader is competence in moving an organization to accomplish its tasks. While successful leaders are invariably respected by those who work with them, they may or may not be liked. Leaders manage activities that accomplish the organization's tasks, and they also manage the human relationships and the emotions generated by participation in those activities. Leaders differ in their relative emphases on tasks and on human relationships. It is very likely that a different mix of emphasis on tasks and on human relationships is required for different organizational purposes and at different stages of an organization's life. The way a leader handles human relationships influences how others feel, whether they like the leader, or whether they experience tension. Leaders do not have to be liked to be effective in accomplishing work tasks. In examining a change process, it is necessary to separate appraisal of the feelings generated by idiosyncratic features of the leader's personality from the leader's effectiveness in moving the organization toward goal attainment.

If Haveliwala's leadership style were plotted on the Managerial Grid (Blake and Mouton 1964), he would probably rank very high on the task-oriented dimension and considerably lower on the people-oriented axis. All speak of him as very firm in his organizational purposes. He relates to his staff primarily in terms of work priorities. He does not engage in small talk, nor does he express much interest in staff members' personal lives. He demands a great deal and rarely rewards others with any expression of personal pleasure or thanks. Some of his staff believe that he views expressions of work-related distress as a weakness, although others recount examples of his sensitive treatment of them at moments of organizational crisis. He undoubtedly has his own moments of anxiety or anger, but he rarely shares his feelings, not even with those staff closest to him.

Although he appears to be a distant and formidable figure, especially to line staff, staff do not seem to fear him. It is important to be in his favor. The worst punishment seems to be that someone falls out of favor. However, all recognize that to gain and retain his favor, one must accomplish organizational purposes. He is absolutely reliable in his commitments and in backing his staff in fulfilling their responsibilities. His staff trust him fully in that regard.

He does not participate very much in clinical work or teaching. He does not visit the wards frequently, nor does he have personal connections with patients or with line staff. He has demonstrated his concern for patients by supporting tangible improvements in patient care, and he is very vigorous in pursuing any hint of patient mistreatment. Staff agree that good patient care is provided, but they say it is because of the staff's concern and not the leader's. The staff experience his pressure for production but not his concern for people.

In consequence of his task orientation, some staff continue to question his affective commitment to Harlem Valley. Some believe that he is motivated by a desire to establish a professional reputation. Some say he is interested in innovations that promote the hospital's and thus the director's personal reputation. This image does not seem to have any detrimental effect on the workings of the institution itself. People are doing their jobs and respond to his leadership.

A strong task orientation and an interest in moving ahead seem characteristic of corporate leaders who sense they have the opportunity to reach the top of the executive ladder. Sensitivity to people may be a bonus, but it is less important to leadership than the competence to get the job done (Kanter 1977). It is also possible that a highly task-oriented style of leadership is essential in changing an organization such as Harlem Valley. A human-relations effort may enable people to feel comfortable with what they are doing and to understand each other, but it may be that a leader's determination to get the job done is the major force that will overcome institutional inertia.

Client Needs and System Needs

Human-service organizations have many goals (Hasenfeld and English 1975). As an open system, a human-service organization engages in resource exchanges with its environment. (A psychiatric center receives tax monies, and in turn it serves people in need, helps solve a community problem, and presumably returns productive citizens to the community.) An open system retains some of the resources it receives for maintainence and for growth. Systems that are highly reactive to variations in the exchange process may direct a considerable portion of their resources toward enhancing the exchange. However, publicly supported human-service organizations obtain their resources only indirectly from exchanges with their environments. They therefore have greater potential for converting those resources to the system's benefit. In this instance, we mean by the system's benefit the use of resources to enhance the working conditions and rewards for employees, rather than the conditions of patients. Ideally, there should be no conflict between patient needs and an organization's needs. In practice, some degree of tension is inevitable (Von Bertalanffy 1968; Katz and Kahn 1966; Schulberg and Baker 1975). In any change process, it is useful to consider how resources are being used for both client needs and system needs.

Harlem Valley commits what appears to be an unusual (for state institutions) portion of its resources to indirect services, to inservice training, and to a variety of staff functions (for example, monitoring, evaluation, and planning) in contrast to line functions (for example, direct patient care). The director has insisted that offices for outpatient facilities be located in good buildings, in desirable locations, and that they be tastefully decorated. The various monitoring devices use personnel time, and, as we have noted, some line staff feel that the extensive elaboration of indirect services and administrative activities have come at the expense of an increased workload for them. Moreover, some of the activities in which it engages may seem like conspicuous consumption. Harlem Valley partially supported a widely advertised conference that included prestigious (and expensive) professional celebrities and public figures. It has invited prestigious, expensive consultants to teach in its inservice programs or to participate in aspects of the development of its programs.

Are these examples of an open system converting resources for its own benefit? One can argue that the presence of prestigious figures as consultants and panelists in inservice education does little more than publicize the institution, and its director to professional leaders. However, Harlem Valley personnel are exposed to leading figures in the field and presumably benefit from those contacts. Such contacts may assist in recruitment. Harlem Valley's ability to offer inservice continuing medical-education credits may well make it easier for the organization to recruit medical staff to its rural location. The director feels his center now has adequate medical staff, although many other psychiatric centers have difficulty in attracting and holding such staff. Its track record of sponsoring outstanding educational programs may well make it easier for the organization to attract outside funds for the support of training programs.

Some see the expenditure of funds for first-class offices as unseemly for a state institution and attribute it to the director's desire to enhance the institution. The director believes that in the past, state services have not been well regarded by the professional community, and it is necessary to overcome that image. Moreover, if personnel are to provide first-class service, they must perceive themselves as first-class citizens within the service community.

Few organizations can demonstrate as much change in as short a time as Harlem Valley. If it appears that monitoring devices and the use of staff time in administrative and executive functions were integral features of the change effort, then it may be that the standards other institutions employ for allocating resources to various functions need to be reexamined. The director and some of his executives argue that clinical services tend to be highly inefficient in most institutions, and their approach improves services by improving efficiency.

Organizational Growth and Development

In any human-service institution, there is always the possibility that resources will be used for purposes of improving conditions of staff, without necessarily contributing to the care of clients. In the early days of the state hospital system, hospital directors were likened to feudal lords. They had palatial homes on hospital grounds and used hospital staff and patients to provide their families and their chief lieutenants with personal services. Today such uses of hospital resources are much more limited. However, directors have power and considerable discretionary authority. It is possible that some resources are employed to provide for the staff, and for the leadership's benefit without consequences for improved patient care. As we have indicated, it is useful to examine Harlem Valley's development from this perspective.

The initiation of new projects is a case in point. The process, while sometimes formal and planned in relation to clearly understood priorities, is also informal and not clearly related to existing service priorities. A new project may sometimes originate informally based on what appears to have been casual shop talk with the director at a cocktail party. The director is a prolific source of ideas, and ready to support innovations that make sense to him. Some of the staff view some of his ideas as wildly impractical and see it as their function not so much to investigate the feasibility of a new proposal, as to "derail" it. (In contrast to the initial steps, the implementation of specific projects seems to have been preceeded by very careful staff work, to judge from some of the program proposals included as addenda to EC minutes.) Is the director using institutional resources to satisfy impulsive, personal whims, or does he have some larger vision of institutional development that he has not yet made clear to his staff?

One of the director's goals is to develop Harlem Valley into an educational center with a strong clinical research arm and with affiliations with outstanding universities and medical schools. In order to achieve that goal, it is necessary to make the center attractive to training institutions. Its innovative community programs are one attraction. However, good programs are not sufficient for an out-of-the-way psychiatric center to develop an affiliation with a pretigious training center. To accomplish its aims, Harlem Valley made the training center the attractive offer of an unusually large sum of money to support some residents and medical-school faculty. The affiliation agreement may provide academic titles for some present Harlem Valley staff. Outside observers, and some Harlem Valley staff, have their reservations about the value of the arrangement.

Another example is instructive. One staff member reported that the director wished to start an art museum and characterized it as another of his "off-the-wall ideas." When the director was asked about it, he said that he had noticed that his hospital had cumulated fifty years' of patient art; that many other hospitals had similar collections; that the collections would be of interest as cultural artifacts, and might have some scientific value; and the idea of patient art might well attract external funding.

In both instances, the director had a long-range aim of enhancing the institution's reputation. In the instance of the training program, the affiliation was presented as part of a plan to bring highly qualified consulting staff to the center, to bring the best residents, and hopefully to attract more highly qualified staff. The consulting staff and the medical school affiliation would upgrade both the service program and the center's public image. Similarly, the purpose of the art museum was to enhance the center's reputation. The director feels that state-supported psychiatric centers are in relatively weak positions to call on the state's resources because the system has tended to serve lower rather than middle-class clientele. He feels the middle class will not freely use the state service system unless it has a reputation for providing the highest quality of care. Enhancing a center's reputation makes it more acceptable to the middle class as a treatment resource and thus builds community and political support for first-class services within the state system.

How should one evaluate the use of institutional resources for training purposes or for the development of an art museum to enhance the center's reputation? One can ask questions about whether the expressed aim of making the psychiatric center acceptable to the middle class is at all a feasible aim, and if it is not feasible, is it an example of an institution's resources being converted to satisfy a leader's whims or the leader's personal creative impulses? Even if the idealistic aim could have been accomplished, does it legitimately fall within the director's prerogatives to pursue vague, long-range aims? To what extent should institutional resources be allocated to the pursuit of such aims, and to what extent should a psychiatric-center director be responsible only for the efficient management of clinical services? Should a psychiatric-center director take on

the responsibility for long-range institutional development and for the development of programs in relation to the community's needs as he or she sees them?
By what standards of value or of accomplishment does one judge one course
against the other? Can a psychiatric-center director within the public system
be a visionary as well as a manager, and if a visionary, what is the proper allocation of resources to the management of the tasks on hand and to making real
images of the future?

Organizational Growth and the Competition for Resources

Just as we can raise questions about the psychiatric-center director's role in
developing community support for the institution's programs, we can also ask
whether he has a role in assessing and fulfilling service and preventive needs in
the community. If the psychiatric center provides a full range of services, then its
requirements for resources increases, and it puts the institution in competition
with others for scarce resources. If other agencies have responsibilities that they
are unable or unwilling to fulfill, does the psychiatric center have a responsibility
to either stimulate others to develop the services or to find the resources necessary to develop the services?

Graziano (1969) has pointed out that human-service agencies tend to
minimize competition among themselves through the allocation of service
territories to each agency. They maintain those boundaries, and those monopo-
lies, by a policy of avoiding "duplication of service." Psychiatric centers within
the state system are not in direct competition with each other. Each has a
designated territory. However, geographic boundaries are not necessarily functional boundaries, and the interaction of psychiatric centers with other service
agencies may well reach across territorial boundaries. Harlem Valley Hospital
is located in a county for which it had no service responsibilities. It is also located near Connecticut and Massachusetts. Should a psychiatric-center director
relate to and use resources outside its geographic boundaries if it makes sense
to do so, or should one be limited by arbitrary political boundaries?

Psychiatric centers are quasi-autonomous units within a larger system, but
as part of a larger system, unusual activity in one part can have effects on other
parts of the system. Psychiatric-center directors have discretionary authority
and within fairly broad limits, can define their own tasks. If one psychiatric-
center director defines the mission differently and acts on that different definition, there may well be implications for others in the system. Has a director who
has acted differently introduced a new competitive element into the system?

In the course of releasing patients to the community, Harlem Valley has
gone outside its catchment area to find nursing-home, and proprietary-home
beds, and family-care sponsors for its patients. The rules governing welfare
payments made it necessary to send patients back to their counties of origin,

even though the chronic patients no longer had ties to their original communities. In 1973 when Harlem Valley was discharging patients to the New York City area, it sent clinical teams out to the city to develop after-care facilities. The territory belonged to another center, but evidently no prior arrangements had been made with the other center to follow the patients. While Harlem Valley mobile clinical teams did follow their patients, a great deal of travel was involved, and it was questionable whether the staff could maintain the mobile service. Eventually Harlem Valley and the other institution reached some understanding about the provision of after-care for its patients, but the agreement came after the fact, when the patient placement was a fait accompli.

Harlem Valley personnel felt they were fulfilling their clinical obligations to their clients by moving them into the community and by providing after-care for them. Even though the return of clients to a distant area outside of Harlem Valley's normal purview was dictated by archaic welfare-law residence requirements, Harlem Valley was affecting another center's area of responsibility. In Harlem Valley's view, nothing would have happened for a long time, if ever, if they had entered into prolonged negotiation with the other center. In Harlem Valley's view, it was acting in the best interests of its patients and in keeping with its mandate to place as many patients into the community as possible. However, in acting that way, it impinged on the responsibilities of another institution. Assuming Harlem Valley's view is correct, that negotiations would have led to interminable delays was its first responsibility to its patients or was it to tacit understandings about how components of a system are to relate to each other?

Within the state system, centers are allocated catchment areas in order to make the provision of services rational. Everyone within the catchment area knows where to go for services. By sending patients into other catchment areas, so the argument goes, Harlem Valley might well have been adding confusion to an orderly system. If all centers related to all catchment areas indiscriminately, chaos would reign. Did the goal of deinstitutionalizing patients justify actions that might have created difficulties for the smooth functioning of the mental-health system?

Similar questions can be raised about the placement of patients in Connecticut and Massachusetts homes, or in nursing homes and proprietary homes in New York State outside of its catchment area. The placements could not have been made without the agreement of social-service departments that paid the bills. Harlem Valley claims that it did not place patients without first ensuring the placement was appropriate and without making arrangements for follow up, for consultation, and for inservice training of personnel. Harlem Valley argues that it took the initiative in searching out appropriate facilities in order to fulfill its clinical responsibilities. If beds were available in other center's catchment areas, it was because the other centers were not making use of these resources.

Others argue that Harlem Valley could not have provided the after-care services that were necessary, and that eventually patient responsibility did fall to them. One can argue that it should not make any difference within a state system, but clearly it does since the allocation of resources on a statewide basis depends on patient load and the delivery of services. One center's activities does have an impact on other centers' workloads and financial resources.

In deinstitutionalizing rapidly and in going outside of its catchment area, Harlem Valley was violating traditional and tacit understandings among psychiatric-center directors that they will not impinge on each other's resources without agreement. (After 1976, at least according to the Harlem Valley's Placement Manual, patients were placed outside of its catchment area only with the receiving center's consent.) Moreover, by deinstitutionalizing rapidly and by developing a variety of community-based services using resources no different from those available to other centers, Harlem Valley may have acted as a pacesetter within the larger New York system, just as we have described some unit chiefs as acting as pacesetters within the Harlem Valley system. If so, Harlem Valley may well have generated competitive tension with the state system, just as tensions were created within its own system. The tensions are less crucial because the various centers do not interact with each other on a day-by-day basis, but their existence may point to a problem in developing cooperation among centers based on functional, rather than arbitrary geographic considerations.

Harlem Valley's director was also aware that if his center were to provide services for patients in communities within his catchment area, he would have to use his center's resources to develop them. Negotiations with community agencies led Harlem Valley executives to the conclusion that community agencies were reluctant to enter the field of providing for chronic patients. Having come to that conclusion, Harlem Valley proceeded to develop its own outpatient and after-care services. It may have been that if Harlem Valley executives and the director had exercised more patience or had adopted more persuasive and conciliatory attitudes toward professionals and officials in local communities, the local communities might have eventually cooperated with Harlem Valley. It is not clear they would have. However, once Harlem Valley entered the field, it quickly expanded its services beyond the provision of care for released chronic patients. On the grounds that it was part of the psychiatric center's mission to provide services to high-risk groups and to prevent hospitalization, Harlem Valley began to provide diverse services targeted to many other patient groups than its own former inpatients.

In so doing, the center put itself in direct competition with county and voluntary agencies serving the same populations. While it may be true that there are more than enough clients for all services and while Harlem Valley can justify its programs in terms of a broader definition of the psychiatric center's mission, there is an organizational self-interest involved as well. The creation of diverse community-based services justifies retention of resources within Harlem Valley's budget. What appears from one perspective to be the fulfillment of an expanded definition of clinical responsibility in keeping with modern concepts of community mental health can from another perspective appear as empire building.

Harlem Valley's director has engaged in political skirmishes with local mental-health authorities about whom shall provide which services. These skirmishes now seem to be settled as Harlem Valley has established itself as a significant provider of services in its communities. However, they leave questions about the role a psychiatric-center director should play in shaping mental-health policies in local communities.

New York State mental-hygiene-legislative policy appears to be one of encouraging local governments to develop appropriate mental-health services—at least that appears to be the thrust of provisions for partial reimbursement of local communities for serving mental patients. The existing legislation contributes to the political skirmishing. While it is built on the hopes of providing better service to clients, as it should be, it does not really recognize the problem that different groups seek fiscal advantage or power and control over resources. It recognizes that there are different service providers, but the legislation has no powerful or coherent provisions for ensuring cooperation. Some of its provisions seem to convey double messages. Local communities are encouraged to take responsibility for planning for their own needs, but the state can tell them what those needs ought to be by withholding approval of plans. Local communities are given responsibility for planning, but they do not control the financial resources for carrying out those plans. The state has control over the resources, and sometimes state facilities have greater apparent freedom to act than do local facilities. Local communities feel their authority is violated when the state facility does not plan with them sufficiently or seems to act in a unilateral fashion in their territory. Given that local private agencies tend to serve one population and the state facilities another, the legislation that designates the local community as the planning body and gives the state mental-health office authority to disapprove plans by withholding funding guarantees some degree of conflict. The existence of skirmishes should lead to a careful study of structural features of the social and political context. While it is easier to think of conflicts as the result of personality clashes, it is unlikely they are.

Harlem Valley's director has actively developed community-based services under state auspices and has lobbied directly and indirectly for legislation to bolster the state's role in outpatient service delivery. What are the responsibilities of psychiatric-center directors? Should center directors remain invisible, keeping their institutions out of the limelight, or should they be active in shaping mental-health policies? What are the implications of different definitions of the role for the development of modern services? What are the implications of different definitions of the role for the system as a whole?

The Diffusion of Innovation

If a psychiatric center shows that it has been able to reallocate its resources so that it does deinstitutionalize without dumping, then its methods are of interest to all other psychiatric centers with the same aim. In contrast to the hard sciences, it is difficult to develop unambiguous evidence of the effectiveness of human-service innovations. It is also difficult to describe key features of a particular context that made an innovation feasible. The human-service field has been influenced by faddish concepts and practices that turned out to have little merit in the long run. Reports of new methods have sometimes presented only initial successes and have glossed over difficulties. Skepticism of claims in the human-service field is always warranted.

Social psychologists tell us that the credibility of a communication depends in part on the credibility attributed to the communicator by listeners. Kanter (1977) points out that because of uncertainties in the task environment, top executives feel most comfortable with people who are like themselves. In this regard, Yoosuf Haveliwala is an unlikely leader. Foreign born and foreign trained, he did his residency and postdoctoral work in provincial settings. He is not an Ivy League product, nor a graduate of one of the major, highly reputed residency programs. He served in the Buffalo Psychiatric Center, which was undergoing a great deal of change, but it was not a major research center. He was deputy director, clinical, at the South Beach Psychiatric Center, one of New York State's showplace facilities, but he did not move on to the directorship of one of the more desirable urban or suburban psychiatric centers, nor to public administration as did some of his South Beach colleagues. He went on to a center that had a relatively poor reputation, and one that was slated to close. On the basis of career trajectory alone, one would not have predicted that Yoosuf Haveliwala would have been the person others would look to for professional leadership. It may be that because he seems an unlikely leader, others will look at his considerable accomplishments with more than a normal amount of skepticism.

He has shown himself to be strong, willing to pursue an independent course of action even when that course violated tradition or created political conflict. He has not always deferred to the wishes of others in the state hierarchy, and he has taken actions that have brought him into conflict with some colleagues in other psychiatric centers. Although some describe his manner in negotiation as forthright, others experience his initial approach as aggressive and abrasive. Although he seems to have been able to work through difficulties with some of those who have been his adversaries in the past, his actions have not made friends for him. He has used administrative prerogative and discretionary authority in creative, but nontraditional ways, and others, more comfortable with conventional approaches, may be concerned about how one could follow such methods without transgressing the bounds of propriety.

Beyond the director's leadership style are other issues. Did Harlem Valley create a community support system, and is there evidence that what it did benefited its patients? To diffuse an innovation that does no good makes no sense. At the time of this study not every element of a fully developed community support system was in place and operative in each part of its catchment area; Harlem Valley executives were the first to admit that.

Search for Change provided residences in but a few of the catchment area's communities. Not every portion of the catchment area had an adequate hospitalization-diversion unit. A vocational placement precisely suitable for each patient was not available. A few of the vocational facilities were rather minimally developed, and although there were some very good facilities, it would be stretching a point to call some of them workshops. Welfare authorities did not always cooperate fully in providing income for released patients, and undoubtedly some struggled with inadequate incomes.

While many of the proprietary and nursing homes did seem to be decent places providing acceptable living conditions, a few were not. Some patients were maintained in less than desirable facilities because no good alternative was available. [See Levine (1979) for a discussion of a similar problem of the dependence of welfare officials on inadequate private facilities as a limit on enforcement of standards earlier in the history of the development of proprietary nursing homes.] Harlem Valley executives attempted to work with proprietors of substandard facilities to improve care, but undoubtedly a diligent investigator would turn up examples of less than the best placements.

Some local communities protested they were being saturated with released patients, and a proprietary home with ex-patients was forced to relocate from a residential neighborhood. The usual stories about former patients urinating in the streets are reported by those who have questions about the value of deinstitutionalization. A search for deficiencies would undoubtedly turn up some.

Harlem Valley claims its patients were benefited. We did not have the resources to undertake an independent evaluation of that claim by conducting systematic follow-ups of patients. We relied on internal reports and published studies and on the credibility of professionals, some of whom were in research rather than operational roles. In addition to the written record and interviews with staff, we undertook to interview Harlem Valley's "enemies," state- and local-government officials and mental-health workers who had had some conflict with Harlem Valley's director and who were competing with its programs.

We were very careful to probe for specifics to pin down complaints about Harlem Valley's services. For example, one official stated that Harlem Valley did not follow its patients into the community. On questioning, he said that he had no personal knowledge, but he referred us to a line mental-health professional who delivered services in that community but who had no affiliation with Harlem Valley. That person informed us that in the early days Harlem Valley did have regular contact with its patients in the proprietary home in question, but later after an agreement had been worked out with another state hospital to assume clinical responsibility for patients who had been placed outside of Harlem Valley's catchment area, they ceased following those patients. It was also his view that the home had been a decent one at first, but the proprietor reneged on promises he had made while recruiting clients for the home.

Yes, Harlem Valley's patients were located in less than fully desirable homes. Yes, Harlem Valley was no longer following those particular patients, but neither of those facts undercuts Harlem Valley's claim that they fulfilled their responsibilities when they were. formally responsible. We followed up on other allegations as well. One official told us of a patient released to a day-care center who had jumped off a railroad bridge and broken both ankles. The official presented the incident as evidence that patients who should not have been released were being released. When asked for another example, the official was at a loss to provide it.

Critics said its services were overstaffed and therefore expensive or that the records of services rendered were inadequate or even inflated. Some services were undoubtedly poorly attended, and one school-based program was discontinued because of a lack of referrals to the program. However, no one disputed claims that they followed patients and provided emergency care and consultation to proprietary homes. Even after a rather lengthy discourse on administrative inadequacies, on lack of political cooperation, on the expense of Harlem Valley's programs, and on the superiority of local programs, without prodding, the critic added that Harlem Valley staff were sincerely concerned with providing humane care to patients. That official could not fault the clinical services per se. He agreed that services for chronic clients were not being provided adequately locally.

Harlem Valley's program-evaluation unit did a one-year follow-up of patients placed in the community. The report treated patients who could not be contacted as unsuccessful placements. However, even with that bias against its own success, the report showed that 72 percent of the patients were still in the community after one year. Of those discharged to nursing homes and other institutions, 91 percent had no rehospitalizations after one year. That record is quite good compared to other facilities. Its program-evaluation reports also showed that its outpatient centers maintained contact for at least the initial months with almost all patients who were discharged.

A published study (Christenfeld and Haveliwala 1978) also established that at least for the sample studied, patients were content with their community placements. The methodology of that study was interesting. A group of student nurses who had expressed serious question about the values of deinstitutionalization were enlisted as participant observers. They were sent out into the community facilities to interview patients and to observe. The report that patients seemed content was based on visits by people who had started out as skeptics. Now it is possible that they were sent to only the best homes and that a systematic sampling would reveal something quite different. Nonetheless, some credible evidence for adequate placement is provided.

As part of the review of documents, we examined the minutes of the monitoring committee that visited community-based facilities. The members of the committees did visit, and they did call deficiencies to the attention of the center's executive committee. The minutes did not reveal the actions taken, but the interviews with individuals who participated produced examples of negotiations with proprietors, and some examples of the discontinuation of the use of a proprietary home that was not up to Harlem Valley's standards. The individuals we interviewed impressed us with their sincerity as well. In other words, the data that were persuasive came from several sources, and the sources complemented each other. Moreover, we could uncover little evidence to the contrary, despite efforts on our part to do so.

In our judgment, Harlem Valley appeared to be providing services at least at the level of the state of the art. If there is benefit to many patients to be supported in the community, then it is our best judgment that Harlem Valley was providing those benefits to its patients. It did so by reallocating its resources and by expanding its treatment facilities. Given good reason to believe that patient care improved, the organizational revitalization at Harlem Valley is a considerable accomplishment worthy of study for what it tells us about the process and the possibilities for organizational change in public agencies embedded within a large bureaucratic structure.

The Harlem Valley experiment in organizational change deserves consideration precisely because it was a planned change. Haveliwala had a plan for change, and he used rather familiar methods. The mix of elements is familiar, but the use of several elements in a coherent whole is unique in the community mental-health literature, the evaluation literature, and the literature on organization and management. Harlem Valley's contribution is the demonstration that familiar methods can be integrated into an organic whole, and when so integrated, predictable results follow.

These elements include a leadership style that blends forthrightness and definiteness of purpose with the open use of data to track progress, leading to public accountability and constructive competition. It includes a deep understanding of the nature of bureaucratic organizations, the willingness to take advantage of flexibility inherent in a large bureaucracy, and the willingness to use discretionary authority to accomplish defined ends.

In addition to understanding how to take advantage of his system, the director looked upon resources creatively. He was willing to "go out of the field," to look for novel solutions to familiar problems, and to implement those solutions. By thinking of resources as flexible and not as fixed and by thinking of people's abilities and not their statuses or formal credentials, the director increased the resource pool and the pool of human talent available to him. He used concrete rewards, but more important, he used the reward that stems from creating opportunities for personal growth and development for those willing to accept the challenge.

The leader's personal style is important to understand. He is highly task oriented, but he is also very clear about his purposes, and he communicates those purposes unambiguously. He also elicits confidence in his leadership because he is competent and resourceful in solving problems. While some may react to a lack of expressions of personal concern, that factor is less crucial than his absolute reliability, his trustworthiness, his consistency, and his demonstrated will to pursue policies he feels are correct, even in the face of opposition and problems. It may be that there was a fortuitous combination of talented people and circumstances enhancing the potential for leadership to accomplish organizational goals. We cannot estimate the relative weights to be assigned to such indeterminate factors. On the other hand, it should be taken as an article of faith that in any organization the size of Harlem Valley, there is a sufficient number of talented individuals who will prove invaluable in carrying out programs, if the leader recognizes their abilities, and provides the organizational climate that encourages creative effort. One need only look beyond formal status and formal credentials.

It is precisely because the elements that went into producing change are familiar that their blend invites study to illuminate the degree to which one can expect that the consistent application of principles will produce replicable results. The Harlem Valley story is important because it provides a concrete example that static organizations need not remain that way, that planned change is possible.

References

Alley, S., and Blanton, J., eds. 1978. *Paraprofessionals in mental health: An annotated bibliography, 1966–1977.* Berkeley, Calif.: Social Action Research Center.

Anderson, D., and Benjaminson, P. 1976. *Investigative reporting.* Bloomington, Ind.: Indiana University Press.

Anthony, W.A. 1979. *The principles of psychiatric rehabilitation.* Amherst, Mass.: Human Resources Development Press.

Anthony, W.A.; Buell, G.J.; Sharratt, S.; and Althoff, M.E. 1972. Efficacy of psychiatric rehabilitation. *Psychological Bulletin* 78: 447–456.

Argyris, C. 1962. *Interpersonal competence and organizational effectiveness.* Homewood, Ill.: Dorsey.

———. 1970. *Intervention theory and method: A behavioral science view.* Reading, Mass.: Addison-Wesley.

Bennis, W.G. 1966. *Changing organizations.* New York: McGraw-Hill.

Bennis, W.G.; Benne, K.; and Chin, R., eds. 1961. *The planning of change.* New York: Holt, Rhinehart and Winston.

Bernstein, C., and Woodward, B. 1974. *All the president's men.* New York: Warner Books.

Bindman, A.J., and Spiegel, A.D., eds. 1969. *Perspectives in community mental health.* Chicago: Aldine.

Blake, R.R., and Mouton, J.S. 1964. *The managerial grid.* Houston, Tex.: Gulf.

Bloom, B.L. 1977. *Community mental health: A general introduction.* Monterey, Calif.: Brooks/Cole.

Bockoven, J.S. 1972. *Moral treatment in community mental health.* New York: Springer.

Bogdan, R., and Taylor, S.J. 1973. *Introduction to qualitative research methods.* New York: Wiley.

Braginsky, B.M.; Braginsky, D.D.; and Ring, K. 1969. *Methods of madness: The mental hospital as a last resort.* New York: Holt, Rinehart and Winston.

Brand, J.L. 1965. The National Mental Health Act of 1946: A retrospect. *Bulletin of the history of medicine* 39: 231–245.

Caplan, R.B. 1969. *Psychiatry and the community in nineteenth-century America.* New York: Basic Books.

Christenfeld, R., and Haveliwala, Y.A. 1978. Patients' views of placement facilities: A participant observer study. *American journal of psychiatry* 135: 329–332.

Comptroller General of the United States. 1977. *Returning the mentally disabled to the community: Government needs to do more.* Washington, D.C.: General Accounting Office.

Connery, R.H.; Backstrom, C.H.; Deener, D.R.; Friedman, J.R.; Kroll, M.; Marden, R.H.; McCleskey, C.; Meekison, P.; and Morgan, J.A. 1968. *The politics of mental health.* New York: Columbia University Press.

Dahl, R.A. 1961. *Who governs?* New Haven, Conn.: Yale University Press.

Demone, H.W., and Harshbarger, D., eds. 1974. *A handbook of human service organizations.* New York: Behavioral Publications.

Deutsch, A. 1949. *The mentally ill in America.* ed. New York: Columbia University Press.

Diesing, P. 1971. *Patterns of discovery in the social sciences.* Chicago: Aldine Atherton.

Douglas, J.D. 1976. *Investigative social research.* Beverly Hills, Calif.: Sage.

Dunham, W.H. 1965. Community psychiatry: The newest therapeutic bandwagon. *Archives of general psychiatry* 12:303-313.

Foley, H.A. 1975. *Community mental health legislation.* Lexington, Mass.: Lexington Books, D.C. Heath and Company.

Gish, L. 1972. *Reform at Osawatomie State Hospital: Treatment of the mentally Ill, 1866-1970.* Lawrence, Kan.: The University Press of Kansas.

Glaser, B., and Strauss, A. 1967. *The discovery of grounded theory.* Chicago: Aldine.

Goffman, E. 1961. *Asylums.* Garden City, N.Y.: Doubleday.

Golann, S.E., and Eisdorfer, C., eds. 1972. *Handbook of community mental health.* New York: Appleton-Century-Crofts.

Goldenberg, I.I. 1971. *Build me a mountain: Youth, poverty and the creation of new settings.* Cambridge, Mass.: MIT Press.

Goplerud, E.N. 1979. Unexpected consequences of deinstitutionalization of the mentally disabled elderly. *American journal of community psychology* 7:315-328.

Gorman, M. 1956. *Every other bed.* Cleveland, Ohio: World Publishing Co.

Graziano, A.M. 1969. Clinical innovation and the mental health power structure: A social case history. *American psychologist* 24:10-18.

Grob, G.N. 1966. *The state and the mentally ill.* Chapel Hill, N.C.: University of North Carolina Press.

_____. 1973. *Mental institutions in America: Social policy to 1875.* New York: Free Press.

Hagedorn, H.J.; Beck, K.J.; Neubert, S.F.; and Werlin, S.H. 1976. *A working manual of simple program evaluation techniques for community mental health centers.* Rockville, Maryl.: National Institute of Mental Health, DHEW Publication (ADM) 76-404.

Hasenfeld, Y., and English, R.A., eds. 1975. *Human service organizations.* Ann Arbor, Mich.: University of Michigan Press.

Heller, K., and Monahan, J. 1977. *Psychology and community change.* Homewood, Ill.: Dorsey.

Henry, J. 1963. *Culture against man.* New York: Random House.

HEW Task Force. 1979. *Report of the HEW task force on implementation of report to the president from the president's commission on mental health.* Washington, D.C.: DHEW Publication No. (ADM) 79–848.

Hollander, E.P. 1978. *Leadership dynamics.* New York: Free Press.

Hollingshead, A.B., and Redlich, F.C. 1958. *Social class and mental illness.* New York: Wiley.

Hornstein, H.A.; Bunker, B.B.; Burke, W.W.; Gindes, M.; and Lewicki, R.J., eds. 1971. *Social intervention: A behavioral science approach.* New York: Free Press.

Hunter, F. 1963. *Community power structure.* Garden City, N.Y.: Doubleday.

Joint Commission on Mental Health and Illness. 1961. *Action for mental health.* New York: Wiley.

Kanter, R.M. 1977. *Men and women of the corporation.* New York: Basic Books.

Katz, D., and Kahn, R.L. 1966. *The social psychology of organizations.* New York: Wiley.

Kiev, A., ed. 1969. *Social psychiatry.* vol. I. New York: Science House.

Koenig, P. 1978. The problem that can't be tranquilized. *The new york times magazine,* 21 May, pp. 14–17, 58.

Lamb, H.R., and Edelson, M.B. 1976. The carrot and the stick: Inducing local programs to serve long term patients. *Community mental health journal* 12:137–144.

Lamb, H.R.; Heath, D.; and Downing, J.J., eds. 1969. *Handbook of community mental health practice.* San Francisco, Calif.: Jossey Bass.

Levine, M. 1979. Congress (and evaluators) ought to pay more attention to history. *American journal of community psychology* 7:1–17.

―――. 1980. Investigative reporting as a research method: An analysis of Bernstein and Woodward's *All the president's men. American psychologist* 35: 626–638.

―――. 1981. *The history and politics of community mental health.* New York: Oxford University Press.

Levine, M., Levine, D.I., and collaborators. 1981. Report of the president's commission on mental health: The development of public policy. *Health Policy Quarterly.*

Likert, R. 1961. *New patterns of management.* New York: McGraw Hill.

Lottman, M.S. 1976. Paper victories and hard realities. In *Paper victories and hard realities: The implementation of the legal and constitutional rights of the mentally disabled,* eds. V. Bradley and G. Clarke. Washington, D.C.: The Health Policy Center, Georgetown University.

McGregor, D. 1960. *The human side of enterprise.* New York: McGraw-Hill.

Marx, A.J.; Test, M.A.; and Stein, L.I. 1973. Extrahospital management of severe mental illness. *Archives of general psychiatry* 29:505–511.

Meyer, N.G. 1974. Legal status of inpatient admissions to state and county mental hospitals. United States, 1972. Statistical Note 105. Washington, D.C.: Division of Biometry, Survey and Reports Branch, NIMH.

Perry, J. 1978. Community placement of chronic psychiatric patients.

Unpublished qualifying paper, Ph.D. Program in Clinical-Community Psychology, SUNY at Buffalo.

President's Commission on Mental Health. 1978. *Report to the president,* vol. I. Washington, D.C.: Government Printing Office.

President's Commission on Mental Health Task Panel on The Nature and Scope of the Problem. 1978. *Report of the task panel.* In Task Panel Reports Submitted to the President's Commission on Mental Health, vol. II. Appendix. Washington, D.C.: Government Printing Office.

Rappaport, J. 1977. *Community psychology. Values, research and action.* New York: Holt, Rinehart and Winston.

Roosens, E. 1979. *Mental patients in town life. Geel—Europe's first therapeutic community.* Beverly Hills, Calif.: Sage Publications.

Rothman, D.J. 1971. *The discovery of the asylum.* Boston: Little, Brown.

Sarason, S.B. 1971. *The culture of the school and the problem of change.* Boston: Allyn & Bacon.

———. 1972. *The creation of settings and the future societies.* San Francisco: Jossey Bass.

Scheff, T.J. 1966. *Being mentally ill.* Chicago: Aldine.

Schulberg, H.C., and Baker, F. 1975. *The mental hospital and human services.* New York: Behavioral Publications.

Stone, A.A. 1975. *Mental health and law: A system in transition.* Washington, D.C.: Government Printing Office.

Szasz, T.S. 1963. *Law, liberty and psychiatry.* New York: Macmillan.

Towbin, A.P. 1969. Self care unit: Some lessons in institutional power. *Journal of consulting and clinical psychology* 5:561–570.

Turner, J.E.; Stone, G.B.; and Tenhoor, W. 1977. The community support program: A draft proposal. Washington, D.C.: Mental Health Services Support Branch, NIMH.

U.S. Senate Subcommittee on Long Term Care. 1976. *The role of nursing homes in caring for discharged mental patients (and the birth of a for-profit boarding home industry).* Supporting paper No. 7. Washington, D.C.: Government Printing Office.

von Bertallanfy, L. 1968. *General systems theory.* New York: George Braziller.

Witkin, M.J. 1979. Provisional patient movement and selective administrative data, state and county mental hospitals, inpatient services by state: United States, 1976. Mental Health Statistical Note No. 153. Washington, D.C.: Division of Biometry and Epidemiology. Survey and Reports Branch, NIMH.

Witten, M.; Kerr, M.; and Turque, C. 1977. State abandons mentally ill to city streets. *Village voice* 22 (31 October) 1, 2, 29.

Wolf, P.C., and Haveliwala, Y.A. 1976. A model for program evaluation in a unitized setting. *Hospital and community psychiatry* 27:647–649.

Zusman, J. 1966. Some explanations of the changing appearance of psychotic patients. In *Evaluating the effectiveness of community mental health services,* ed. E.N. Gruenberg. New York: Milbank Memorial Fund.

Index of Names

Index of Subjects

About the Author

Murray Levine is professor of psychology and director of the Clinical/Community Graduate Training Program in Psychology at the State University of New York at Buffalo. Previously, he directed the graduate program in clinical psychology. at Yale University and worked in its Psychoeducational Clinic. He is a diplomate in clinical psychology of the American Board in Professional Psychology, and in 1977-1978, he served as president of Division 27, Community Psychology, of the American Psychological Association. He is author or co-author of five books, including *Psychology in Community Settings* (with Seymour Sarason and others), *A Social History of Helping Services* (with Adeline Levine), and *The History and Politics of Community Mental Health.*